Neuromuscular Pathology Made Easy

Neuromuscular Pathology Made Easy

Edited by
Maher Kurdi, MD, FRCPC, EFN
Assistant Professor of Neuropathology
Neuromuscular Pathologist
Department of Pathology
Faculty of Medicine in Rabigh
King Abdulaziz University
Kingdom of Saudi Arabia

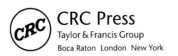

CRC Press
Taylor & Francis Group
Boca Raton London New York

CRC Press is an imprint of the
Taylor & Francis Group, an **informa** business

First edition published 2021
by CRC Press
6000 Broken Sound Parkway NW, Suite 300, Boca Raton, FL 33487-2742

and by CRC Press
2 Park Square, Milton Park, Abingdon, Oxon, OX14 4RN

© 2021 Taylor & Francis Group, LLC

CRC Press is an imprint of Taylor & Francis Group, LLC

This book contains information obtained from authentic and highly regarded sources. While all reasonable efforts have been made to publish reliable data and information, neither the author(s) nor the publisher can accept any legal responsibility or liability for any errors or omissions that may be made. The publishers wish to make clear that any views or opinions expressed in this book by individual editors, authors, or contributors are personal to them and do not necessarily reflect the views/opinions of the publishers. The information or guidance contained in this book is intended for use by medical, scientific, or health-care professionals and is provided strictly as a supplement to the medical or other professional's own judgment, their knowledge of the patient's medical history, relevant manufacturer's instructions, and the appropriate best-practice guidelines. Because of the rapid advances in medical science, any information or advice on dosages, procedures, or diagnoses should be independently verified. The reader is strongly urged to consult the relevant national drug formulary and the drug companies' and device or material manufacturers' printed instructions, and their websites, before administering or utilizing any of the drugs, devices, or materials mentioned in this book. This book does not indicate whether a particular treatment is appropriate or suitable for a particular individual. Ultimately it is the sole responsibility of the medical professional to make his or her own professional judgments, so as to advise and treat patients appropriately. The authors and publishers have also attempted to trace the copyright holders of all material reproduced in this publication and apologize to copyright holders if permission to publish in this form has not been obtained. If any copyright material has not been acknowledged please write and let us know so we may rectify in any future reprint.

Except as permitted under U.S. Copyright Law, no part of this book may be reprinted, reproduced, transmitted, or utilized in any form by any electronic, mechanical, or other means, now known or hereafter invented, including photocopying, microfilming, and recording, or in any information storage or retrieval system, without written permission from the publishers.

For permission to photocopy or use material electronically from this work, access www.copyright.com or contact the Copyright Clearance Center, Inc. (CCC), 222 Rosewood Drive, Danvers, MA 01923, 978-750-8400. For works that are not available on CCC please contact mpkbookspermissions@tandf.co.uk

Trademark Notice: Product or corporate names may be trademarks or registered trademarks and are used only for identification and explanation without intent to infringe.

ISBN: 9780367634278 (hbk)
ISBN: 9780367557263 (pbk)
ISBN: 9781003119135 (ebk)

Typeset in Berling LT Std
by KnowledgeWorks Global Ltd.

Part I General

Part II Muscle

Ahmad Abuzinadah, MD
King Abdulaziz University,
Jeddah, Saudi Arabia

Ahmed Bamaga, MD
King Abdulaziz University,
Jeddah, Saudi Arabia

Ashraf Dallol, PhD
King Abdulaziz University,
Jeddah, Saudi Arabia

Habib Bin Attiah, BSc
King Abdulaziz Medical City,
Jeddah, Saudi Arabia

Fawaz Musa, MSc
King Abdulaziz University,
Rabigh, Saudi Arabia

Neuromuscular pathology is considered a relatively new evolving subspecialty. Over the last decade, a wealth of information about muscle diseases with remarkable advances at both the histological and genetic aspects has considerably improved the ability to evaluate patients with myopathy. Some studies have already prompted new classifications and strategies, and some are under elucidation.

This book, *Neuromuscular Pathology Made Easy*, is particularly aimed at neurologists, neuropathologists, trainees, and medical students involved in clinical neuroscience and pathology. I made a huge effort to bring this treasure completely up-to-date. It is accompanied by large amounts of scientific data previously available from a great variety of sources. The intent of this book is to provide both a clinical and histological manual that presents information about common and rare neuromuscular diseases in a simplified, integrated, and rapidly accessible format. In keeping with this goal, the text is combined with many simple illustrations and tables so all readers can find an easy access or approach to the diagnosis.

This book also provides a concise outline with practical tips to facilitate proper histopathological diagnosis.

The material is divided into three sections: general, muscle and nerve. Each section is divided into chapters. The first section deals with basic principles of neuromuscular histology and physiology, processing technique, and laboratory management. It also provides muscle and nerve templates for final diagnostic reports. The second and third sections deal with neuromuscular diseases that are summarized in a stepwise approach, with algorithms and organized tables. Illustrations and descriptions of muscle pathology are arranged in color-coded boxes with particular emphasis. Tables and algorithms summarize each disease based on definition, genetic association, clinical features, electrophysiological findings, and myopathological features.

I hope this book conveys some of the excitement of these advances whilst integrating them into practical accounts of current principles of complete neuromuscular diagnosis.

Maher Kurdi

ACKNOW   rS

Special thanks to my family, who have graciously tolerated the time spent at home on this book. My thanks also to the histopathology technicians and photographers for their valuable contribution to this work. Many special thanks to our neuromuscular team at King Fahd Medical Research Center at King Abdulaziz University. I also have been supported by an excellent editing team, especially Samantha Cook and Rebecca Edwards, whose expertise is demonstrated in the beautiful layout of this handbook.

ABC	Avidin–biotin complex
ACH	Acetylcholine
ADD	Autosomal dominant disease
ADP	Adenosine diphosphate
ALS	Amyotrophic lateral sclerosis
AMP	Adenosine-5-monophosphoric acid
AMPD	Amyoadenylate deaminase
ANM	Autoimmune necrotizing myopathy
ANO5	Anoctamin 5
APOA	Apolipoprotein-A
ARD	Autosomal recessive disease
ATP	Adenosine triphosphate
ATPase	Adenosine triphosphates
AZT	Azidothymidine
BAG3	Bcl-2-associated athanogene
BMD	Becker muscular dystrophy
BOOP	Bronchiolitis obliterans pneumonia
BSA	Bovine serum albumin
CBM	Cytoplasmic body myopathy
CD	Cluster of differentiation
CK	Creatine kinase
CLL	Chronic lymphocytic leukemia
CMAP	Compound muscle action potential
CMD	Congenital muscular dystrophy
CMTS	Charcot–Marie–Tooth syndrome
CMV	Cytomegalovirus
CoA	Coenzyme A
COX	Cytochrome c oxidase
CPT	Carnitine palmitoyl transferase
CRE	Cytochrome c reductase
CSF	Cerebrospinal fluid
CV	Conduction velocity
CVD	Collagen vascular disease
DAG	Dystrophin-associated glycoprotein
DM	Myotonic dystrophy
DMD	Duchenne muscular dystrophy
DMPK	Myotonic dystrophy protein kinase
DMVP	Dermatomyositis vascular pathology
DUX4	Double homeobox protein 4

ECG	Electrocardiogram
EDD	Emery-Dreifuss dystrophy
EGR-1	Early grow response protein-2
EM	Electron microscopy
EMA	Epithelial membrane antigen
EMG	Electromyogram
ESR	Erythrocyte sedimentation rate
ETFA	Electron transfer flavoprotein
FAP	Familial amyloid polyneuropathy
FCMD	Fukuyama muscular dystrophy
FDH2	Flavin adenine dinucleotide
FF	Fresh frozen
FFPE	Formalin-fixed paraffin embedded
FHL1	Four-and-half-LIM domain 1
FKRP	Fukutin-related protein
FPBM	Fingerprint body myopathy
FSHD	Facioscapulohumeral dystrophy
GAN	Giant axonal neuropathy
GBE1	Glucan branching enzyme
GBS	Guillain–Barre syndrome
GSD	Glycogen storage disease
GSN	Gelsolin protein
GT	Gomori trichrome
GVHD	Graft-versus-host disease
GYS1	Glycogen synthetase 1
H&E	Hematoxylin and eosin
HIV	Human immunodeficiency virus
HMG	Hydroxy-methyl-glutaryl
HMSN	Hereditary sensorimotor neuropathy
HNRNP	Heterogeneous nuclear protein
HPP	Hypokalemic periodic paralysis
HPS	Hematoxylin-phloxine-saffron
IBM	Inclusion body myositis
ILD	Interstitial lung disease
Jo-1	tRNA synthetase
KSS	Kearns–Sayre syndrome
KU	Speckled nuclear
LAMP	Lysosomal associated protein

LDH	Lactate dehydrogenase
LDL	Low density lipoprotein
LEM	LAP2-Emerin-MAN1
LFB	Luxol fast blue
LGMD	Limb-girdle muscular dystrophy
LS	Leigh syndrome
MAC	Membrane attack complex
MAD	Myoadenylate deaminase
MERFF	Myoclonic epilepsy ragged fibers
MFM	Myofibrillar myopathy
MH	Malignant hyperthermia
MHC-I	Major histocompatibility complex I
MHCf	Myosin heavy chain fast
MHCn	Myosin heavy chain fetal/neonatal
MHCs	Myosin heavy chain slow
MitDNA	Mitochondrial DNA
MLPA	Multiplex ligation probe amplification
MNGC	Multinucleated giant cell
MR	Mental retardation
MRI	Magnetic resonance imaging
NAD	Nicotinamide adenine dinucleotide
NAIP	Neuronal apoptosis inhibitory protein
NAM	Necrotizing autoimmune myopathy
NBT	Nitroblue tetrazolium
NCT	Nerve conduction test
NGS	Next generation sequencing
NMJ	Neuromuscular junction
NML	Neuromuscular lab
NPD	Niemann-Pick disease
NRM	Nemaline rod myopathy
OCTN	Organic cation transporter
OMIM	Online Mendelian Inheritance in Man
OPMD	Oculopharyngeal muscular dystrophy
ORO	Oil red O
PABPN1	Polyadenylate-binding protein
PAN	Polyarthritis nodosa
PAS	Periodic acid-Schiff
PCR	Polymerase chain reaction

PFK	Phosphofructokinase
PGAM	Phosphoglycerate mutase
PGBD	Polyglucosan body disease
PGFK	Phosphoglycerate kinase
PTAH	Phosphotungstic acid hematoxylin
RA	Rheumatoid arthritis
RBF	Ragged blue fibers
RER	Rough endoplasmic reticulum
RIIM	Regional ischemic myopathy
RRF	Ragged red fibers
rRNA	Ribosomal RNA
RSMD	Rigid spine muscular dystrophy
RYR1	Ryanodine receptor 1
SAE	Small ubiquitin-like modifier activating enzyme
SDH	Succinate dehydrogenase
SEPN1	Selenoprotein N1
SLE	Systemic lupus erythematosus
SLONM	Sporadic late-onset rod myopathy
SMA	Spinal muscular atrophy
SMCHD	Structural maintenance hinge domain
SMN	Survival motor neuron
SNAP	Sensory nerve action potential
SNHL	Sensorineural hearing loss
SR	Sarcoplasmic reticulum
STIM1	Stromal interaction molecule-1
SYNE-1	Synaptic nuclear envelope protein-1
TAM	Tubular aggregate myopathy
TFI	Tubulofilamentous inclusion
TIF	Transitional intermediary factor
TNPO3	Transportin-3
TRI	Tubuloreticular inclusion
TRIM32	Tripartite-motif containing gene 32
tRNA	Transfer RNA
TTR	Transthyretin
VCLAD	Very long-chain dehydrogenase
VCP	Valosin-containing protein
WDM	Welander distal myopathy
WES	Whole exome sequencing

WGS	Whole genome sequencing
WWS	Walker–Warburg syndrome
XLR	x-linked recessive
ZASP	Z-line alternatively spliced protein
ZNF9	Zinc finger protein-9

PART I
GENERAL

CHAPTER 1
MUSCLE AND NERVE HISTOLOGY

Contents

1.1 Muscle Histology

Muscle tissue is differentiated into smooth, cardiac, and skeletal muscles. This differentiation embryonically starts to develop from mesoderm during the 7th week of gestation and it completely forms by the 28th week of gestation. The nuclei take their peripheral positions after 20 weeks of gestation. Skeletal muscle is elongated on longitudinal sections and striated in cross section. The entire portion is enclosed in a connective tissue sheath called *epimysium*, which is composed of extracellular matrix and irregular collagens. The epimysium connects into the tendon sheath and divides the muscle into groups of bundles, or fascicles, separated from each other by perimysium (**Figure 1.1**). The myotendinous junction area sometimes mimics dystrophy (pseudomyopathy), as it may show alternative features of hypertrophic and atrophic fibers, excess fibrous tissue, and multiple internal nuclei (**Figure 1.2**).

Each group of muscle fascicles is composed of uniform muscle fibers called *myocytes*. They are separated from each other by a network of reticular fibers and extracellular matrix, called *endomysium*.

Each muscle fiber contains either a single nucleus or multiple nuclei and a cytoplasm called *sarcoplasm*, and it is surrounded by a plasma membrane called *sarcolemma*. The nuclei are usually peripherally located, heterochromatic, and containing fine nucleoli and stippled nucleoplasm. They stain blue with hematoxylin and red with Gomori trichrome. Centrally positioned nuclei for more than 3% of a whole fascicle is considered abnormal.

The sarcoplasm contains multiple organelles including mitochondria, sarcoplasmic reticulum, Golgi apparatus, microtubules, glycogens, ribosomes, lipid droplets, and myofibrils. The mitochondria are located at the level of the

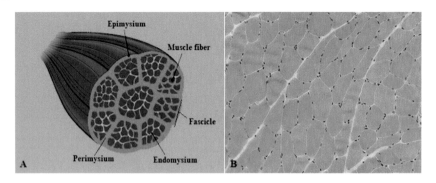

Figure 1.1 **(a)** An illustrated photograph of skeletal muscle layers. **(b)** Cross section of normal skeletal muscle shows the muscle fibers within the fascicles. (H&E ×20.)

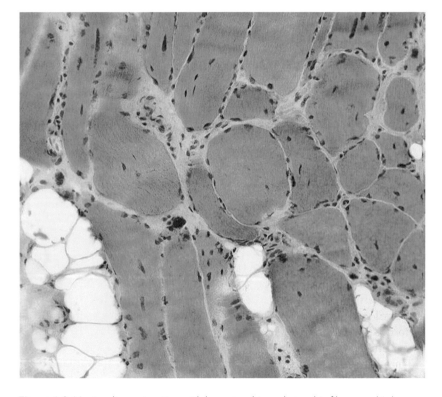

Figure 1.2 Myotendinous junction with hypertrophic and atrophic fibers, multiple internal nuclei, and increased connective tissue. (H&E ×40.)

Table 1.1 Intracellular and extracellular sarcolemmal proteins associated with each muscle fiber.

Protein	Structure	Interaction site
Dystrophin	Sarcolemmal protein with four domains (actin-binding, central rod, carboxyl terminus, cysteine-rich domain)	Sarcoglycan, dystroglycan syntrophin, dystrobrevin
Sarcoglycan	Transmembrane protein that has four subtypes: α, β, γ, δ	Dystrophin, filamin-C
Dystroglycan	Transmembrane protein (α, β). α-II laminin (merosin)	Dystrophin, caveolin-3
Dysferlin	Type II transmembrane protein	Caveolin-3
Caveolin-3	Protein found in caveolae	Dysferlin, RYR1
Myotilin	Sarcomeric Z-disc protein	Filamin-C, α-actinin
Emerin	Nuclear membrane protein anchored to cytoskeleton	Actin, lamin A/C, CTNNB1

Abbreviations: RYR1: ryanodine receptor 1; CTNNB1: catenin beta-1 protein.
Note: The interaction site is the binding site where each protein interacts with another one.

I-band. They present in type I fibers more than type II fibers, but this is not considered a consistent distinguishing feature.

The sarcolemma consists of an inner plasma membrane (plasmalemma) and outer membrane (external basal lamina). The plasmalemma is an excitable membrane composed of a lipid bilayer and a variety of ion channels and proteins present on the cytoskeleton. Some of these sarcolemmal proteins are summarized in **Table. 1.1** and **Figure 1.3**.

The plasmalemma extends deeps into the muscle fibers, forming T-tubules that carry the depolarization of action potential inside the fibers. Hence, a T-tubule with two terminal cisterns forms a triad. The triad has a voltage-gated calcium channel and ryanodine receptor. T-tubules and sarcoplasmic reticulum are essential components involved in muscle contraction.

The main functional units of each muscle fiber are myofibrils. Each myofibril is composed of bundles of myofilaments that are aligned precisely to form sarcomere in longitudinal section. Each sarcomere extends between two Z-lines and is composed of two bands; A-band dark and I-band light (**Figure 1.4**). These bands are associated with myofilaments. The myofilaments are subdivided into:

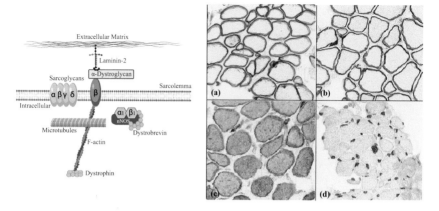

Figure 1.3 (*Left*) A diagram of sarcolemmal muscle proteins. (*Right*) Groups of important muscle proteins: **(a)** dystrophin; **(b)** sarcoglycan; **(c)** dysferlin; **(d)** emerin (×40). This figure was created with Biorender.com.

1. **Thin filaments** (7 nm in diameter) consist of a protein called F-actin, which originates at the Z-line at the level of the I-band. Actin is attached to other proteins such as myotilin, filamin, and tropomyosin.
2. **Thick filaments** (15 nm in diameter) consist of a protein called myosin, which originates at the H-desk at the level of the A-band. The A-band is bisected by the M-line.

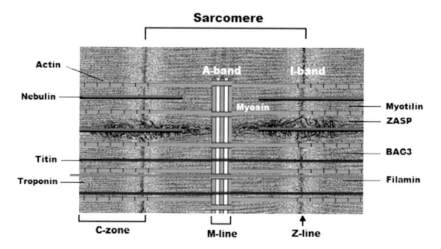

Figure 1.4 A diagram of sarcomere and muscle proteins. A-band is bisected by M-line while I-band is bisected by Z-line.

The structural organization of myofibrils is maintained by titin, α-actinin, and nebulin proteins. These proteins are present in the Z-line interacting with other proteins that are associated with varieties of neuromuscular disease. These proteins include telethonin; myozenin; filamin-C; Z-band alternatively spliced, PDZ-motif (ZASP); and four and a half LIM domains protein 1 (FHL1).

Intramuscular nerves, capillaries, and muscle spindles are found between muscle bundles.

1.1.1 Mitochondria

Mitochondria are double-membrane structures located in the sarcoplasm adjacent to the I-band (**Figure 1.5**). These "powerhouses of the cell" make up energy and are involved in several cellular functions including glycolysis, amino acid metabolism, fat oxidation, calcium homeostasis, and cell death apoptosis.

Each mitochondrion structurally consists of outer and inner membranes. The inner membrane is rich in cardiolipin and folded to form cristae, which makes it highly impermeable to ions, electrons, and proteins. Unlike the outer membrane, the inner membrane does not contain porins. Both membranes share "contact sites" to exchange proteins and molecules. Additionally, a large number of protein complexes called *respiratory chains* are present in the

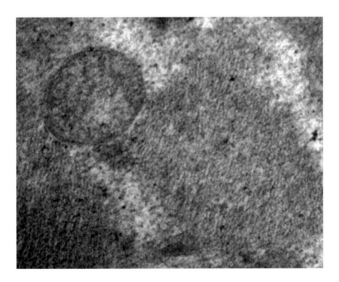

Figure 1.5 An electrograph ultrastructural section of sarcoplasm showing the mitochondria (500 nm).

inner membrane surface. Each respiratory chain is composed of the following enzymes:

- Complex I: Nicotinamide adenine dinucleotide (NADH)
- Complex II: Succinate dehydrogenase (SDH)
- Complex III: Cytochrome C reductase (CCR)
- Complex IV: Cytochrome C oxidase
- Complex V: ATP synthase

These enzyme complexes form the electron transport chain (ETC), which is responsible for the transfer of electrons along the chain, and function as proton pumps.

Mit-DNA comprises 16,569 base pairs in length and encodes 37 maternally inherited genes including two copies of ribosomal-RNA genes, 22 transfer-RNA genes, and 13 protein-coding genes.

Within the matrix space, the enzymes facilitate the process of glycolysis to produce pyruvate and acetyl-CoA and help in the subsequent oxidation of these intermediates in the Krebs cycle. Called *oxidative phosphorylation*, this process is responsible for ATP production.

1.2 Peripheral Nerve Histology

Peripheral nerves develop in the fetus during the 15th week of gestation. Each nerve trunk is divided into multiple fascicles. Each individual fascicle consists of three layers (**Figure 1.6**):

1. *Epineurium*, the outer layer, is a dense collagenous connective tissue containing thick elastic fibers.
2. *Perineurium*, the middle layer, is a cylindrical fibrocollagenous layer containing epithelial membrane antigen (EMA) positively stained perineurial cells. Renault bodies are normal structures with ellipsoid shapes located in the sub-perineurial space. They contain fibroblasts and mast cells and lack of axons. Of 600 sural nerve biopsies, 2% have Renault bodies. Unfamiliarity with these bodies' appearance may result in diagnostic errors. They could be misinterpreted as endoneurial edema or an infarct.
3. *Endoneurium*, the inner layer, is a loose connective tissue that surrounds individual nerve fiber (axons), fibroblasts, mast cells, fixed macrophages, and capillaries. The endoneurium is completely isolated from the perineurium and Schwann cells.

Axons arise from the cell body at axon hillocks where the thin dendritic process extends. Each axon is surrounded by a plasma membrane called

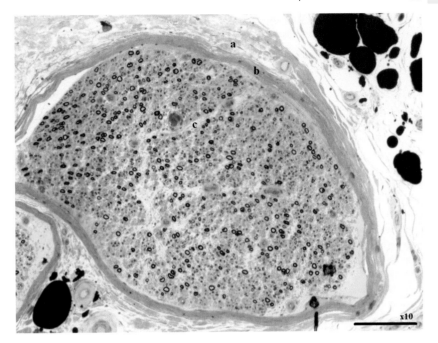

Figure 1.6 An Epon-embedded cross section of peripheral nerve (×10) shows three layers: **(a)** epineurium, **(b)** perineurium, and **(c)** endoneurium. The endoneurium contains myelinated and non-myelinated axons. (Reprinted with the permission of Dr. Ahmad Abuzinadah, King Abdulaziz University.)

axolemma and contains nuclei and axoplasm; the latter has no ribosomes or rough endoplasmic reticulum (RER). The axolemma forming the myelin sheath is referred to as *myelinated axon*. Axons lacking myelin sheaths are called *unmyelinated axons* or *Remak fibers*. The myelinated axon (1–20 μm in diameter) is longer than the unmyelinated axon (0.2–2 μm in diameter). The unmyelinated fibers are always multiple, sensory, and characterized ultrastructurally by the presence of a single basal lamina surrounding the entire fiber. In the sural nerve, the ratio of myelinated to unmyelinated fibers is 1:4.

Schwann cells are nucleated spindle cells that envelope axons and serve as electrical conductors. They contain Golgi apparatus, few mitochondria, and scattered inclusions called *Reich granules*. These granules contain lipid or Elzholz bodies that should not be mistaken as abnormal inclusions. The continuity of the myelin sheath is interrupted at regular intervals by nodes of Ranvier.

Table 1.2 Normal age-related changes in the peripheral nerve.

- Increase in collagen thickness of endoneurium
- Reduced myelin densities
- Duplication of endothelial capillaries
- Minimal axonal degeneration or regeneration
- *Scattered Reich granules*

Table 1.2 shows age-related changes in the peripheral nerve that should not be misdiagnosed as cellular abnormalities.

References

Blake DJ, Martin-Rendon E. Intermediate filaments and the function of the dystrophin-protein complex. Trends Cardiovasc Med. 2002; 12(5): 224–228.

Gao Q, McNally E. The dystrophin complex: structure, function, and implication for therapy. Compr Physiol. 2015; 5(3): 1223–1239.

Luther PK. The vertebrate muscle Z-disc: sarcomere anchor for structure and signalling. J Muscle Res Cell Motil. 2009; 30: 171–185.

Matsuda C, Hayashi YK, Ogawa M, et al. The sarcolemmal protein dysferlin and caveolin-3 interact in skeletal muscle. Hum Mol Genet. 2001; 10(17): 1761–1766.

Matsuda C, Kiyosue K, Nishino I, et al. Dysferlinopathy fibroblasts are defective in plasma membrane repair. PloS Curr. 2015; 7.

Meier C, Bischoff A. Polyneuropathy in hypothyroidism. Clinical and nerve biopsy study of 4 cases. J Neurol. 1977; 215: 103–114.

Michele DE, Campbell KP. Dystrophin-glycoprotein complex: post-translational processing and Dystroglycan function. J Biol Chem. 2003; 278(18): 15457–15460.

Pette D, Staron RS. Myosin isoforms, muscle fiber types, and transitions. Microsc Res Tech. 2000; 50: 500–509.

Pina-Oviedo S, Ortiz-Hidalgo C. The normal and neoplastic perineurium: a review. Adv Anat Pathol. 2008; 15: 147–164.

Rando TA. The dystrophin-glycoprotein complex, cellular signaling, and the regulation of cell survival in the muscular dystrophies. Muscle Nerve. 2001; 24(12): 1575–1594.

Takahashi J. A clinicopathologic study of the peripheral nervous system of the aged: sciatic nerve and autonomic nervous system. Geriatrics. 1966; 21: 123–133.

Whiteley G, Collins RF, Kitmitto A. Characterization of the molecular architecture of human caveolin-3 and interaction with the skeletal muscle ryanodine receptor. J Biol Chem. 2012; 287(48): 40302–40316.

MUSCLE AND NERVE FIBERS CLASSIFICATION

Contents

2.1 Muscle Fiber Classification

Skeletal muscle is composed of a mixture of fibers that differ in their physiological and chemical properties. This differentiation is important in clinical practice as it is considered an early tool used in the histopathological approach. By using the enzymatic histochemistry technique, practitioners can differentiate muscle fibers into two types; type I and II fibers. Type II muscle fibers are subcategorized into IIa and IIb. This precise differentiation is established based on several factors including oxidative and glycolytic activities, as described in **Table 2.1**.

It sometimes is difficult to differentiate type I fibers from type II fibers using hematoxylin and eosin (H&E) stain. However, oxidative enzymes and other histochemistries may help. It is now widely accepted that most neuromuscular labs use myosin heavy chain isoforms rather than using adenosine triphosphatase (ATPase) to differentiate between fiber types. In contrast to ATPase, myosin isoforms can detect regenerating and immature fibers as well as fibers in postmortem muscle. Antibodies to *slow* myosin heavy chain show type I fibers darker than type IIa/IIb fibers (**Figure 2.1**), whereas antibodies to *fast* myosin heavy chain show type II fibers darker. ATPase is carried out in different pH concentrations (4.3 and 9.4). ATPase with pH 4.3 shows type I fibers darker than type II fibers.

All oxidative enzymes, including NADH, COX, and SDH, highlight type I fibers darker than type II fibers. This is because type I fibers contain more mitochondria than type II fibers.

The proportion of each muscle fiber type varies between each body muscle. Knowing the site of muscle biopsy is important in assessing the muscle fiber types. For example, deltoid and biceps muscles have a proportion of type I fibers higher than quadriceps muscles. This also applies to individual muscle

Table 2.1 Main features of different types of skeletal muscle fibers.

	Type I	Type IIa	Type IIb
Color	Dark	Light	
Mitochondria	Rich	Poor	
Twitch speed	Slow	Fast	
Fatigability		Resistant	Sensitive
Capacity	Highly oxidative		Highly glycolytic
ATPase pH 4.3	+++	+	–
ATPase pH 9.4	+	+++	+++
NADH-TR	+++	++	+
COX	+++	++	+
SDH	+++	++	+
Phosphorylase	+	+++	+++
PAS	+	+++	+++
Oil-red	+++	+	+
Ab to slow myosin	+++	+	+
Ab to fast myosin	+	+++	+++

Abbreviations: ATPase: adenosine triphosphatase; NADH: reduced nicotinamide adenine dinucleotide-tetrazolium; COX: cytochrome C-oxidase; SDH: succinate dehydrogenase; PAS: periodic acid-Schiff; Ab: antibodies.

fibers close to the quadriceps. The tibialis anterior has predominant type I fibers compared to the quadriceps muscle which has predominant type II fibers. The fiber type predominance should also be differentiated from fiber type grouping seen in denervation. Fiber type grouping always affects type I fiber and is associated with other histological features of the neuropathic process.

Chapter 7 explains the basic biochemical characteristics of each muscle enzyme and labeling on cellular morphology.

2.2 Peripheral Nerve Fiber Classification

Nerve fibers are functionally segregated into sensory afferent fibers and motor efferent fibers. This classification is important in physiological studies and when assessing nerve damage. When the axon is crushed, the axonal degeneration process occurs in the part of the axon away from the cell body. This is known as *Wallerian degeneration.*

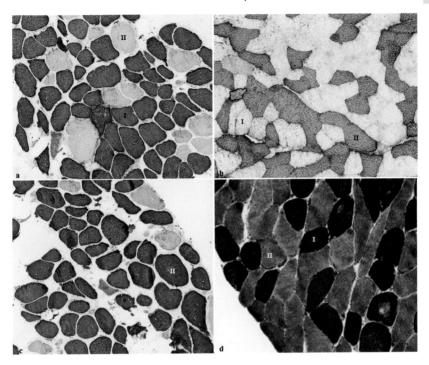

Figure 2.1 Muscle fiber classification. **(a)** *Slow* myosin heavy chain shows dark type I fibers and light type II fibers. **(b)** *Fast* myosin heavy chain shows the opposite staining of *slow* myosin with dark type II fibers and light type I fibers. **(c)** Type II fiber predominance. **(d)** NADH can classify muscle fibers with type I fibers darker than type II fibers.

Based on their diameter and conduction velocity (CV), nerve fibers are also subclassified into A, B, and C types (**Figure 2.2**). A-type is subdivided into alpha, beta, gamma, and delta fibers. This classification is known as Erlanger and Gasser classification. The CV is considered the main cutoff factor in this classification, which depends on the extent of nerve myelination. In myelinated fibers, depolarization initiates faster than in unmyelinated fibers. Therefore, the CVs in group A myelinated fibers are higher than group B and C fibers (**Table 2.2**). These changes can be detected only during electrophysiological studies. The pathological changes associated with these abnormal fibers can be detected by examining the nerve fibers themselves.

The teased-fiber technique is the best approach for studying peripheral nerve fibers. It assesses the nerve fiber diameter, myelin segment size, and the pathologic changes affecting the internodes or the paranodal regions. This obsolete technique is no longer performed nowadays, but it is sometimes

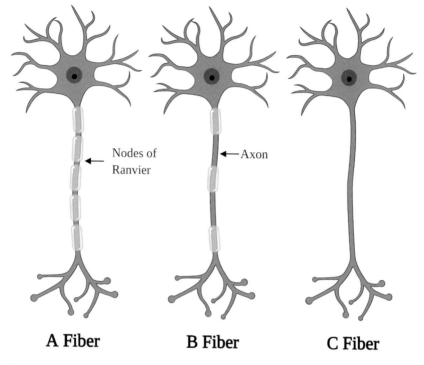

Figure 2.2 Peripheral nerve fiber classification. This figure was created with Biorender. com.

Table 2.2 Peripheral nerve classification.

Type	Diameter (μM)	Myelination	CV (m/sec)	
Group A	2–20	Myelinated	12–120	
Alpha	Extrafusal muscle			
Beta	Intrafusal muscle and skin touch and pressure			
Gamma	Intrafusal muscle and proprioception			
Delta	Pain and temperature sensation			
Group B	0.4–1.2	Myelinated	3–15	Preganglionic fibers
Group C	*0.3–1.3*	*Unmyelinated*	*0.7–2.3*	*Postganglionic fibers*

helpful during nerve damage or demyelinating diseases. The examining nerves should be 10 mm long and stained for 24 hours in Sudan black stain. The nerves are separated into smaller fiber bundles on a glass slide. Changes, when present, can usually be recognized during the preparation, in particular, segmental demyelination and axonal degeneration.

References

Brooke MH, Kaiser KK. Muscle fiber types: how many and what kind? Arch Neurol. 1970; 23: 369–379.

Johnson MA, Polgar J, Weightman D. Data on the distribution of fibre types in thirty-six human muscles. An autopsy study. J Neurol Sci. 1973; 18: 111–129.

Krinke GJ, Vidotto N, Weber E. Teased-fiber technique for peripheral myelinated nerves: methodology and interpretation. Toxicol Path. 2000; 28(1): 113–121.

Whitwam JG. Classification of peripheral nerve fibers. An historical perspective. Anaesthesia. 1976; 31(4): 494–503.

CHAPTER 3

CLINICAL NEUROPHYSIOLOGY

Ahmad Abuzinadah, MD

Contents

Neurophysiological evaluation is considered an extension to patient symptoms and signs in clinical practice. It includes two essential electrodiagnostic (EDx) tests. The patient is evaluated first with nerve conduction study (NCS) followed by electromyography (EMG). Both studies are important in neuromuscular biopsy interpretation. They are also specifically essential in the diagnosis of neuropathy or myopathy, or for patients presenting with coexisting features.

The three major objectives of EDx evaluation are summarized as the following:

1. To localize the pathological lesion within the peripheral nervous system (**Table 3.1**). The following are the possible localizations that EDx can confirm:
   a. Anterior horn cell.
   b. Nerve roots.
   c. Plexus.
   d. Polyneuropathy, which is further categorized by EDx into:

      – Length-dependent distal neuropathy.
      – Non-length-dependent polyneuropathy and polyradiculoneuropathy.

   e. Sensory ganglionopathy
   f. Mononeuropathy, which is further categorized by EDx into:

      – Compression and focal neuropathy.
      – Mononeuritis multiplex.

g. Neuromuscular junction (NMJ), which is further categorized by EDx into:

- Presynaptic NMJ disorders.
- Post synaptic NMJ disorders.

h. Muscle diseases.

2. Pathophysiology of a nerve injury: EDx can differentiate between axonal and demyelinating neuropathy (**Table 3.2**).
3. Pathophysiology of a muscle injury: EDx can differentiate between two major types of myopathy:

- Irritative myopathy such as inflammatory myopathies or muscular dystrophies; usually shows fibrillations and positive sharp wave potentials (**Table 3.3**).
- Non-irritative myopathy such as congenital myopathy; usually has no fibrillations and positive sharp wave potentials (**Table 3.3**).

Specific diagnostic clues:

- Myotonia is associated with myotonic dystrophy or myotonia congenita and Pompe disease.
- Fasciculation is associated with motor neuron diseases.
- Myokymia is associated with radiation plexopathy.

3.1 Nerve Conduction Study (NCS)

NCS measures the conduction within the nerve in response to electrical stimulus. In the motor portion of the nerve, the nerve trunk is stimulated by electrical volts or amperes and the response of the motor fibers is recorded indirectly by the electrical action potentials generated in the muscle fibers. The response is recorded through electrodes placed over the muscle and is depicted as a waveform (**Figure 3.1**). This waveform is called *compound muscle action potential* (CMAP). CMAP represents a summation of all muscle fiber action potentials, and it has certain characteristics such as latency, amplitude, and conduction velocity (CV). Impairment of a certain property may give a clue toward the diagnosis (**Table 3.2**). Examples of commonly recorded motor nerves include: median, ulnar, common peroneal, and tibial nerves.

In the sensory portion of the nerve, the nerve trunk is stimulated by electrical volts or amperes and the response is recorded by electrical stimulus placed over the pure sensory distal branch of the nerve. The response is depicted in waveform (**Figure 3.1**). This waveform is called *sensory nerve action potential* (SNAP), and it also has certain properties such as peak latency, amplitude,

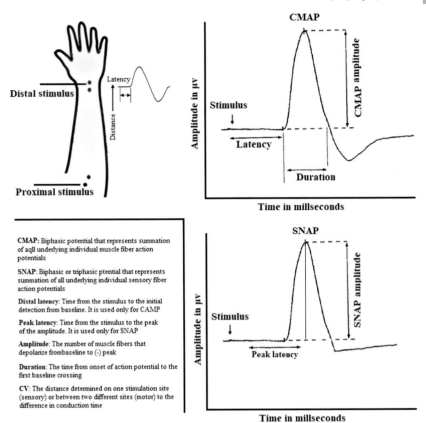

Figure 3.1 Compound muscle action potential (CMAP) and sensory nerve action potential (SNAP) in electrophysiological diagnostic tests.

and CV. Examples of commonly recorded sensory nerves include: median, ulnar, superficial peroneal, and sural nerves.

3.2 Electromyography (EMG)

This test records the electrical activity within the specific diseased muscle. It evaluates the motor unit action potential (MUAP), which is the number of motor units activated during muscle contraction. MUAP can be described in terms of the duration, amplitude, phases, stability, and firing characteristics of the abnormal muscle.

Table 3.3 outlines the abnormal changes seen in EMG in common neuromuscular disorders.

Table 3.1 Patterns of indicative localizations in peripheral nerve.

Localization	Diseases	Electrodiagnostic clues
Anterior horn cell	Amyotrophic lateral sclerosis Spinal muscular atrophy	• Normal SNAP • Small CMAP amplitude • EMG: active and chronic denervation in non-nerve and non-root distribution
Nerve roots	Radiculopathy	• Normal SNAP • May be small CMAP amplitude • EMG: active and chronic denervation in root distribution only • Paraspinal muscle denervation
Plexus	Brachial neuritis Lumbosacral plexopathy	• Small SNAP amplitude • Small CMAP amplitude • EMG: active and chronic denervation in certain trunk or cord distribution • Normal paraspinal muscle on EMG
Non-length-dependent polyneuropathy	Guillain–Barre syndrome Chronic inflammatory demyelinating neuropathy (CIDN)	• Small SNAP amplitude • Small CMAP amplitude • Absent F waves • EMG: active and chronic denervation in proximal and distal muscles
Sensory ganglionopathy	Anti-Hu Sjogren's syndrome	• Absent SNAP • Normal CMAP • Normal EMG
Length-dependent distal neuropathy	Diabetic neuropathy	• Small SNAP amplitude • May be small CMAP amplitude • F waves likely normal • EMG: active and chronic denervation in distal muscles only

Table 3.1 Patterns of indicative localizations in peripheral nerve.
(Continued)

Localization	Diseases	Electrodiagnostic clues
Compressive mononeuropathy	Carpal tunnel syndrome Common peroneal neuropathy at the knee	• Slow conduction velocity in single nerve distribution across compressive/ entrapment sites • Conduction block across compressive/entrapment sites
Mononeuritis multiplex	Vasculitic neuropathy	• Low SNAP and CMAP in multiple nerves, not all of them adjacent to each other • >50% in SNAP or CMAP amplitude in side-to-side comparison • Neurogenic pattern in EMG
Presynaptic NMJ disorders	Lambert–Eaton syndrome Botulism	• >100% increment on fast RNS (>30Hz)
Postsynaptic NMJs	Myasthenia gravis	• Decrement on slow RNS (<5Hz)
Muscle	Inflammatory myopathies Muscular dystrophy Congenital myopathy	• Normal SNAP • Probably normal CMAP • Myopathic in EMG

Abbreviations: SNAP: sensory nerve action potential; CMAP: compound muscle action potential; EMG: electromyography; RNS, repetitive nerve stimulation; neuromuscular junction (NMJ).

Table 3.2 Demyelinating versus axonal neuropathy in NCS.

	Demyelinating neuropathy	Axonal neuropathy
Amplitude	Slightly reduced at early stage	Markedly reduced
Latency	Marked prolongation	Slight prolongation
Conduction velocity	Marked slowing	Slight slowing
Conduction block	Could be seen	Not seen
Temporal dispersion	Could be seen	Not seen
F-waves	Delayed latency or absent	Not affected
H-reflex	Absent or delayed	Not affected

Table 3.3 Electromyography interpretation.

Pattern	Findings
Neurogenic pattern	• Late recruitment • Large MUP amplitude • Wide motor unit duration • Polyphasia
Myopathic pattern	• Early recruitment • Small MUP amplitude • Short MUP duration • Polyphasia
Activities	
Active denervation	Fibrillations PSW Fasciculation CRD
Irritative myopathy	Fibrillations, PSW, and CRD

Abbreviations: MUP: Motor unit action potential; PSW: positive sharp waves; CRD: complex repetitive discharge

References

Amato A, Russel JA. Neuromuscular disorders. McGraw-Hill Medical, New York. 2008.

Daube JR. AAEM minimonograph #11: needle examination in clinical electromyography. Muscle Nerve. 1991; 14: 685–700.

Preston DC, Shapiro BE. Electromyography and neuromuscular disorders: clinical electrophysiological correlations. Elsevier, London; New York. 2013.

CHAPTER 4

NEUROMUSCULAR LABORATORY

Neuromuscular pathology service is passionately committed to providing a specialized assessment for the most comprehensive and contemporary diagnosis of neuromuscular diseases in adult and pediatric patients. This service should be presented in a functional, precise lab unit. The laboratory handling of muscle and nerve biopsies is specific and requires specialist knowledge beyond that of routine anatomical pathology services. Without a specialized NML, clinicians would have difficulties diagnosing challenging neuromuscular cases. Indeed, a fully equipped lab dealing with muscle and nerve tissue specimens is essential.

The equipment provided in a NML is somewhat distinct from other specialized lab equipment. In addition to the general equipment and instruments found in any histopathology lab, an extensive panel of special instruments, chemicals, stains, enzymatic reactions, immunoperoxidase staining for muscle proteins, and electron microscopy facilitate the diagnosis of all myopathies, dystrophies, and peripheral neuropathies.

An NML can be established in a single adequately ventilated room inside any generalized histopathology laboratory with excellent safety and workable stations (**Figure 4.1**). A 9.0 m² room is enough space to establish a lab, aided with fume and ventilation safety hoods (**Figure 4.2**). The room space must be divided into specialized areas, and each area should have its own precautions. Our lab at King Abdulaziz University (King Fahd Medical Center) has two benches—one is a workable station for initial muscle procedures, and the other is used for cutting and staining. The rotary frozen machine (cryostat) is placed in a separate corner. The cryostat should be switched on 1–2 hours before starting any biopsied muscle tissue processing.

The stored chemicals and nitrogen liquid are dangerous materials, and they must be placed a few walked-meters from the working station. A well-trained technician, having the knowledge to deal with muscle and nerve specimens, is essential.

The following equipment or instruments are essential to establish an NML:

- Rotary cryostat with power cord, heat extractor, low-profile coated knives, and cork desk (e.g., Leica CM1860UV) (**Figure 4.3**).

23

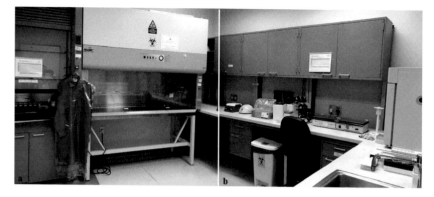

Figure 4.1 Neuromuscular lab unit: Dr. Kurdi's lab at King Fahd Medical Center, Roya, King Abdulaziz University.

- Analytical balance, magnetic stir bars, incubator, and pH meter.
- Freezer (–80°C) and cryogenic liquid nitrogen tank and base.

Other devices for barcode printing and patient sample labeling are mandated to preserve patient identification. Barcode label printers are available from several manufacturers. Because the muscle or nerve pieces are received frozen and segmented, paraffin-associated tissue processing technology (e.g., tissue processor for embedding, trimmer, or surgical microtome) is not usually

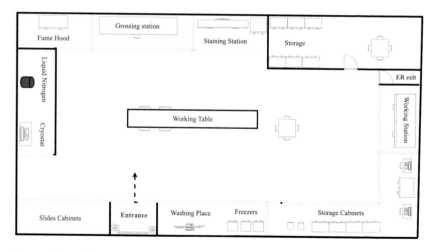

Figure 4.2 An illustrated diagram of a neuromuscular lab. The lab can be established in a single adequately ventilated room provided with essential equipment.

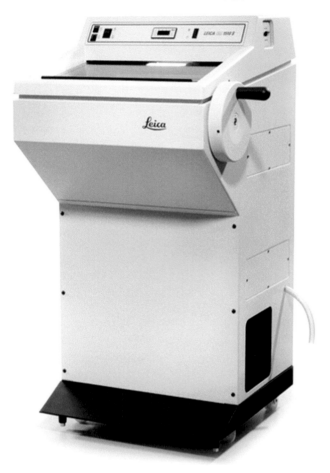

Figure 4.3 Rotary cryostat from Leica. Used to cut frozen muscle, the cryostat is considered the main essential device in the lab. (*The illustrated cryostat machine belongs to our NML.*)

required in the NML. However, the tissue processor in the general pathology lab can be used when paraffin-embedded samples are needed. Paraffin-embedded sections are sometimes preferred during nerve biopsy processing using Luxol fast blue (LFB) or silver impregnation stains.

Table 4.1 outlines the essential equipment, instruments, and materials required in a specialized NML.

Table 4.1 Neuromuscular lab essential equipment, instruments, and materials.

Device or instrument	Manufacturer	Model
Barcode label printer	Intermec	PC43d
Rotary cryostat with knife and holder	Leica	CM1860UV
Cryogenic liquid nitrogen, tank, base, and hose	MVE Lab	MVE LAB 30
Dental wax	Canemco Inc.	312
Tragacanth	Sigma	Any
Analytical balance	Fisher Scientific	Mettler PC 2000
Magnetic stir bars	Fisher Scientific	14-513-76
Stirring hotplates	Fisher Scientific	11-497-6A
pH meter	Fisher Scientific	AB15 Plus
Thermal flask (1 L)	Thermo Fisher Scientific	2122
Pipette pump (10 ml capacity)	VWR	53502-233
Eppendorf pipette and tips (0.02–1.0 ml)	Fisher Scientific	Any
Aluminum beaker	VWR	AA39046-KT
Freezer (–80°C)	Non-specific	Any
Staining rack set	Non-specific	Any
Superfrost Plus (+ charged slides) 25×75×1 mm	Fisher Scientific	Any

Note: The manufacturers and models mentioned in this table represent the ones we use in our NML.

CHEMICAL MATERIALS USED IN THE LAB

Chemical materials used in the preparation of muscle and nerve samples are considered essential contents in any NML dealing with tissue processing. These materials are available in the market with different options and a variety of sources and brands. Safely storing chemicals in the lab requires diligence and careful consideration. Because some of these materials are hazardous, they should be stored in a separate closed site provided with enough safety and ventilation precautions. A technical specialist should be trained carefully to handle and store these materials to minimize explosion risks.

Proper personal protective equipment (PPE) must be available. At a minimum, this should include appropriate chemical-resistant gloves and eye protection, and a lab coat. Caution must also be taken during the transport of these materials. Volatile toxics and odoriferous chemicals must be stored in a ventilated cabinet; flammable liquids must be protected in a liquid storage cabinet for this purpose.

Because most muscle histochemical stains require concise manual preparation, the availability of chemical liquids in close proximity to the lab is substantial. Thus, each enzymatic or histochemical reaction has its own preparatory protocol. (See *Chapter 7.*) Every NML in any institution has its own policy and manual, but the practical procedures are always fixed in any protocol. The variability in liquid volumes and tube sizes is flexible.

Chemical materials used in the lab are classified under three categories:

1. *Materials used in the manual preparation of muscle histochemistry* (**Table 5.1**) such as hematoxylin and eosin (H&E) stain, Gomori trichrome (GT), periodic acid-Schiff (PAS), oil red, Congo red, and oxidative enzymatic reactions. These materials are prepared by the technologist specialist following a fixed formulated protocol. Our manual protocol is described in Chapter 7.
2. *Materials used in the preparation of muscle immunohistochemistry.* These materials are ready-to-use antibody kits, manufactured by several companies (such as Leica), and prepared by the technologist via automated immunostainer (such as Ventana). These antibody kits have fixed expiration dates and require system detection kits

Table 5.1 Chemical materials and solutions used in the manual preparation of muscle histochemistry.

Chemical material	Manufacturer
Glacial acetic acid 0.2%	ACP
Adenosine-5-monophosphate	Sigma
Adenosine-5-triphosphate disodium salt hydrate	Sigma Aldrich
Ammonium hydroxide 28%	ACP
Calcium chloride dihydrate	Sigma
3,3-Diaminobenzidine tetra HCL hydrate	Sigma
5,5-Dimethyl 1,3-cyclohexanedione (Dimedone)	Aldrich
Glucose 1-phosphate	Sigma
Nitrotetrazolium Blue chloride	Sigma
Potassium cyanide	Fisher Scientific
Potassium iodide	Fisher Scientific
Propylene glycol	Fisher Scientific
Sodium nitrite	Fisher Scientific
Sodium phosphate dibasic	Sigma
Sodium phosphate monobasic	Fisher Scientific
Sodium phosphate monobasic monohydrate	Sigma
Hydrochloric acid	ACP
Tris (hydroxymethyl) aminomethane	Fisher Scientific
2-Methylbutane	ACP
Catalase from bovine liver	Sigma
Cytochrome C from horse heart	Sigma
β-Nicotinamide adenine dinucleotide reduced disodium hydrate	Sigma
Sodium succinate	Sigma
Trichrome stain LG solution	Sigma-Aldrich
Hematoxylin	Sigma-Aldrich
Eosin Y 515, alcoholic	Leica
Ethanol	Leica
Chloroform	Fisher Scientific
Iodine	Fisher Scientific
Xylene	Chaptec
Pararosaniline base	Sigma
Periodic acid	A&C
Tissue-Tek OCT Compound	Somagen
Ringer lactate	Sigma
Congo red kit	Fisher Scientific

Table 5.1 Chemical materials and solutions used in the manual preparation of muscle histochemistry. (Continued)

Oil red O	Sigma
Schiff reagent	Abcam
Acid phosphatase assay kit	Bio-Optica
Glycogen	Bio-Optica
Formaldehyde 37%	Sigma-Aldrich

and bulk fluids to run them in the immunostainer. **Table 5.2** lists the antibodies commonly used in neuromuscular diagnosis. Many of these antibodies are used to diagnose muscle dystrophy diseases such as dystrophinopathies, sarcoglycanopathies, and dysferlinopathy. Major

Table 5.2 Antibodies (prepared material kits) used in the preparation of muscle immunohistochemistry.

Staining kit with the code	Manufacturer
Myosin Heavy Chain *slow* NCL-MHCs	Leica
Myosin Heavy Chain *fast* NCL-MHCf	Leica
α Sarcoglycan (adhalin) NCL-a SARC	Leica
β Sarcoglycan NCL b-SARC	Leica
δ Sarcoglycan NCL g-SARC	Leica
δ Sarcoglycan NCL d-SARC	Leica
α Dystroglycan NCL a-DG	Leica
β Dystroglycan NCL b-DG	Leica
Dysferlin NCL (Hamlet 1)	Leica
Dystrophin *rod domain* NCL-DYS 1	Leica
Dystrophin *c-terminus* NCL-DYS 2	Leica
Dystrophin *n-terminus* NCL-DYS 3	Leica
β-Spectrin NCL-SPEC1	Leica
Calpain-3 NCL CALP-2c4	Leica
Emerin NCL-emerin	Leica
Merosin (Laminin α2) MAB-1924	Millipore
Caveolin-3 NCL-CAV	Leica
Utrophin NCL-DRP2	Leica
Collagen Type IV	Biotechnology
Major Histocompatibility Complex-MHC class 1 W6/32	Santa Cruz-Abcam
Membrane Attack Complex MAC C5b-9	Dako
P62	Santa Cruz

histocompatibility stain (MHC) is another commonly used antibody in pathological practice that helps in the diagnosis of inflammatory myopathy subsets. Further details about these stains are described in Chapter 7.

3. *Materials used in the preparation of nerve tissue and electron microscopy* (Table 5.3).

Table 5.3 Materials used in the preparation of histochemistry and epoxy-embedded sections of the nerve.

Chemical material	Manufacturer
Acid fuchin	Anachemia
Alpha-terpineol	Fisher Scientific
Aniline blue	Fisher Scientific
Citric acid	Anachemia
Ferric ammonium sulfate	Anachemia
Lithium carbonate	Fisher Scientific
Luxol fast blue (LFB)	BDH
Nitric acid "concentrated"	Anachemia
Phosphomolybdic acid	Anachemia
Picric acid	Sigma-Aldrich
Ponceau xylidine	Chroma-Gesellschaft
Silver nitrate	Fisher Scientific
Sodium thiosulfate	A&C

References

Bancroft JD, Stevens A. The theory and practice of histological techniques, 3rd edition. Churchill Livingstone, Edinburgh. 1990.

Lojda Z, Gossrau R, Schiebler TH. Enzyme histochemistry. Springer Verlag, Berlin. 1979.

Pearse AGE. Histochemistry: theoretical and applied, 3rd edition. Churchill, London. 1968.

CHAPTER 6

BIOPSY PROCESSING PROTOCOL

Habib Bin Attiah and Maher Kurdi, MD

Contents

6.1 Muscle

6.1.1 Selection of Muscle

Muscle biopsy is the initial step of the diagnostic process in a patient with a neuromuscular condition. Accurate selection of the biopsied muscle will help the pathologist to detect and conclude the morphological findings. This is based on a detailed clinical history, physical examination, and investigations of the symptomatic patient. Electrodiagnostic studies through electromyography (EMG) or nerve conduction tests (NCTs) are always helpful in the differential diagnosis as well as the histological assessment.

In general, the main indication of muscle biopsy is a symptomatic patient with evidence of progressive muscle weakness, chronic muscle cramps, or muscle symptoms associated with systemic diseases. Indeed, every muscle biopsy can be a confirmatory tool for electrophysiological findings but unnecessary to confirm a specific diagnosis. In this case, a patient may suffer from other co-existing systemic diseases affecting the muscles or the patient's family may suffer from unknown hereditary myopathic disease that may not show histological findings in muscle biopsy.

To select a good muscle for a biopsy, the following criteria should be taken into consideration:

■ The muscle should not be severely affected by the disease process.

- The previous muscle biopsy site or the site where it had a previous traumatic injury must be avoided, as these sites may show fibrosis and degenerative change.
- The site where the muscle will be taken should not be close to the myotendinous junction nor close to an area rich in fat. Some clinicians use ultrasound to help them identify a muscle free of fat or scarring.

Most biopsies are performed on proximal muscles of the upper limbs, such as deltoid and biceps muscles, or in the lower limbs such as quadriceps muscles (vastus lateralis). In rare cases, tibialis anterior, hamstring, or extensor digital muscles are selected. The pathologist should not neglect the muscle site during microscopic interpretation as some muscles vary with their fiber type distribution. (See *Chapter 2*.)

6.1.2 Muscle Biopsy Surgical Options

For decades, muscle biopsy was commonly performed through open surgical excision under local or general anesthesia. This practice changed in 1861. An alternative option to perform a localized needle biopsy became a common rout, not because it is safer and less time-consuming, but because patients prefer this option. A Bergstrom needle with a sliding cannula should be inserted into the muscle while the other hand holds the thigh. The window is opened by sliding the cannula while the muscle is gently squeezed to slide into the window of the needle. The needle can be reintroduced multiple times through the same incision, if necessary. An average tissue fragment of 0.5–1.0 cm size is enough for tissue processing. It is better to orient the tissue specimen. The muscle should either be kept in an empty container or on a moist saline gauze, ready to transfer to the lab (**Figure 6.1a**).

6.1.3 Muscle Specimen Preparation

The specimen containing muscle shank should be received from the operating room on a moist saline Teflon gauze. This is to ensure the specimen has the ideal integrity, so it is not dried or overly saturated with saline. However, adding any chemical or liquid materials to the container may damage the muscle tissue.

Once the sample is received at the NML, the length and diameter of the muscle piece must be recorded for quality assurance. The specimen should be verified and labelled with patient's identification. At this time, one-third of an aluminum beaker should be filled with 2-methylbutane and then placed in a thermal flask surface touching the liquid nitrogen from the bottom. This step will facilitate an early partial cooling of 2-methylbutane on the flask surface.

The sample usually includes two or three muscle fragments; one is selected to be snap-frozen while the other two fragments are sectioned by 1–2 mm

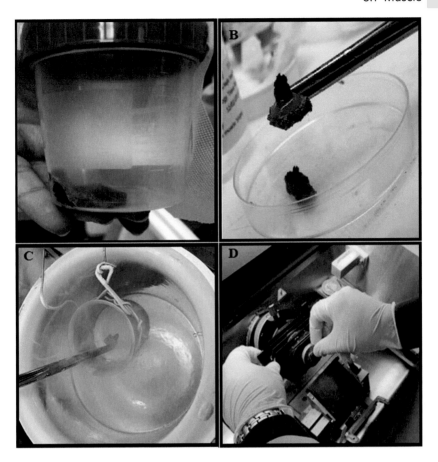

Figure 6.1 Muscle biopsy processing at the lab. **(a)** A surgically excised muscle piece placed in an empty container. **(b)** Mounting the muscle tissue over Tragacanth gum on a Teflon block. **(c)** The Teflon block is immersed in the aluminum beaker containing 2-methylbutane for 20 seconds. **(d)** The muscle block is anchored into the cryostat cork desk to prepare it for sectioning.

and immediately fixed in 10% formalin for paraffin embedding and 3% glutaraldehyde solution for electron microscopy processing. If any muscle fragments remain, they are placed in a cryogenic vial or snap-frozen in liquid nitrogen to be kept in a freezer at −80°C for the future. Some labs place the remaining tissue in an RNA Tube for genetic testing when needed.

The selected frozen fragment is prepared for cross sectioning in a cryostat machine. Loose ends are trimmed to make the fragment as square as possible for sectioning. To embed the muscle, Tragacanth gum is used. The Tragacanth gum is applied to the Teflon block where the muscle fragment is anchored slightly to it (**Figure 6.1b**). The Teflon block serves as a place to secure the muscle fragment and also to provide a solid rigid medium to manipulate it for the flash freezing process.

Using forceps, the technologist immediately immerses the Teflon block into the precooled aluminum beaker containing 2-methylbutane for 20 seconds (**Figure 6.1c**). It is then submerged inside the flask that contains liquid nitrogen for 3 hours. Next, it is cut in the cryostat. This process must be done with the muscle fragment as longitudinal straight as possible. The cross section can be obtained later during tissue cut in the cryostat.

Cryostat sectioning of the muscle fragment is performed when the block reaches an equalized temperature of −30°C. After the block gets fixed in the cryostat clamp, the fragment is sectioned at 6 to 9 μm thickness, using the external rotator (**Figure 6.1d**). During the cut, the glass slide should be approximated to the cryostat knife after serial cutting and trimming.

The glass slides can later be left at room temperature until routine staining applies. Hematoxylin and eosin (H&E) and Gomori trichrome (GT) stain are always the initial routine preparations. The pathologist can initially look at these two slides and decide if additional stains are required (**Figure 6.2**). Several tissue cuts on unstained slides can be performed early in

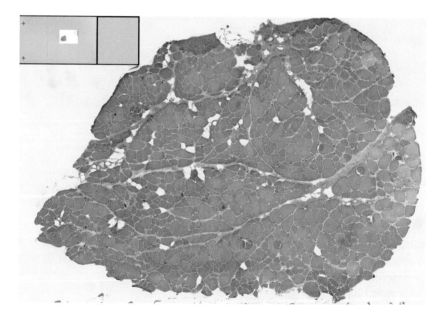

Figure 6.2 Low-power magnification of a muscle biopsy tissue stained with H&E, ready for histopathological assessment.

the procedure and stored in a −20°C freezer until they are ready for staining. Special histochemistry, such as periodic acid-Schiff (PAS) or oxidative enzymatic reactions, should be done on Superfrost slides. (See *Chapter 7*.)

The following is the routine panel of muscle histochemistry:

- H&E and modified GT
- Metabolic stains: PAS and Oil red
- Fiber distribution stains: adenosine triphosphatase (ATPase) with different pH concentration or myosin heavy chain isoforms (*slow* and *fast*)
- Oxidative enzymatic stains: NADH, COX, SDH, and combined COX-SDH stain
- Some labs perform esterase and Congo red as routine stains

6.2 Nerve

6.2.1 Nerve Selection

Because nerve biopsy is rare in clinical practice, its indication has not been delineated. Clinicians ask sometimes for nerve biopsy either because of under diagnosed peripheral neuropathy or a previous unremarkable muscle biopsy but dense clinical features of nerve disease. Some clinicians request a nerve biopsy when there is a question of diagnosis if denervation atrophy is detected in both muscle and nerve biopsies. Asbury et al. emphasized that nerve biopsies in asymmetric and multifocal neuropathies are useful in cases of distal symmetrical polyneuropathies, whether subacute or chronic, axonal or demyelinating features are detected. It is estimated that nerve biopsy could reveal essential information in about 20% of cases and be helpful in a further 20%. It has always been found that chronic inflammatory demyelinating polyneuropathy (CIDP) cannot be ruled out via nerve biopsy only. This means that nerve biopsy has little clinical value in interpreting common polyneuropathic diseases.

Nevertheless, several institutions around the world still use nerve biopsy to assist in diagnoses, although there are no rigid criteria for nerve biopsy indications. When a clinician reaches the point where all clinical and electrophysiological tests fail to diagnose a case, a nerve biopsy is then strongly indicated.

Determination of the nerve biopsy site is always the point of interest. Similar to muscle biopsy, the surgeon should avoid areas where previous surgery or trauma has occurred. Consequently, motor nerves are generally not suitable sites for biopsy as their injury may cause muscle weakness following the procedure. The distal nerve is always preferred, because in most neuropathies the longest fibers are severely affected. Because sural nerve conduction studies are routinely performed in most laboratories, the sural nerve is by far the most common biopsy site. Other nerves such as common peroneal nerves and obturator nerves are also potential sites.

6.2.2 Nerve Specimen Preparation

Nerve specimen preparation is a quite different from muscle sample preparation, as liquid nitrogen is not used in the nerve processing technique. A properly processed nerve biopsy must include resin-embedded semi-thin sections (treated with toluidine blue stain) and ultra-thin sections for electron microscopy. A well-trained technologist should be available to perform the nerve sectioning.

For optimal processing, a segment of 2 cm length of nerve tissue is preferred. Once the sample is received from the operating room, the length and diameter of the tissue should be recorded, and the sample should also be registered for patient identification. Extreme care must be taken when handling the unfixed nerve to avoid crush artifact of the myelin sheath.

Immediately after removal of the biopsy specimen, the fresh nerve is gently straightened on a piece of tongue depressor and wrapped in a piece of gauze moistened with normal saline in a specimen container. The nerve is dissected, using a sharp razor, into three equal parts. The first part is submitted, as a longitudinal section, in a cassette that is immersed inside 10% formalin. The second part is bisected and submitted as cross sections in another cassette immersed in 10% formalin. The last part is dissected into smaller pieces, 1 mm thick longitudinal and cross sections, and submitted in a cassette that is immersed in 3% glutaraldehyde. A portion of it can be processed for teased fiber technique while the remaining parts must be processed for resin-embedding sectioning with epoxy toluidine technique. This technique is considered the best method to read the nerve biopsy specimen.

The nerve is cut with ultra-microtome at 1 μm (semi-thin sections) for the optical microscope and ultra-thin sections for the electron microscope.

The first two portions are processed through a routine paraffin-embedding procedure for staining with H&E. Other special stains that may be performed are Congo red, Luxol fast blue (LFB), modified Bielschowsky, and Masson trichrome. All these stains are used to evaluate myelination, axonal degeneration, and intracellular and extracellular material deposition. Immunohistochemistry for neurofilament stain can also be done to detect axonal changes.

References

Asbury AK, Gilliatt RW. The clinical approach to neuropathy. In: Asbury AK, Gilliatt RW (eds) Peripheral nerve disorders. A practical approach. Butterworths, London. 1984; pp 1–20.

Brockmann K, Becker P, Schreiber G, et al. Sensitivity and specificity of qualitative muscle ultrasound in assessment of suspected neuromuscular disease in childhood. Neuromuscul Disord. 2007; 17: 517–523.

Edwards R. Percutaneous needle-biopsy of skeletal muscle in diagnosis and research. Lancet ii. 1971: 593–595.

Edwards R, Round J, Jones D. Needle biopsy of skeletal muscle: a review of 10 years' experience. Muscle Nerve. 1983; 6: 676–683.

Heckmatt J, Moosa A, Hutson C. Diagnostic needle muscle biopsy: a practical and reliable alternative to open biopsy. Arch Dis Child. 1984; 59: 528–532.

Henriksson KG. Semi-open muscle biopsy technique: a simple outpatient procedure. Acta Neurol Scand. 1979; 59: 317–323.

Neundorfer B, Graham F, Engelhartdt A, et al. Postoperative effects and value of sural nerve biopsies: a retrospective study. Eur Neurol. 1990; 30: 350–352.

HISTOCHEMISTRY PROTOCOL

Fawaz Musa, MSc and Maher Kurdi, MD

Contents

After the biopsy procedure and tissue processing, the neuromuscular tissue is ready for histochemical staining. The staining must be performed on Superfrost charged slides to obtain a good quality and also to maintain the tissue viability on the slides for long periods of time. In *Chapter 4* and *Chapter 6*, we listed the chemical materials used in the preparation of the muscle and nerve specimens as well as the essential histochemistry labeling that we routinely use in muscle pathology practice. We also listed the immunohistochemistry antibodies that help in the differential diagnoses of muscle dystrophy diseases.

In this chapter, we describe the manual technical procedures that the technologist should follow to prepare the histochemical stains. The theoretical background and interpretation of this staining and variations to the staining techniques will also be discussed.

7.1 Histochemical Reaction

The most important stain routinely used in neuromuscular pathology is hematoxylin and eosin (H&E), which clearly visualizes the general structure of the tissue in relation to the fibers, sarcolemmal contents, and the presence of inflammation or other intracellular abnormalities. Histopathological abnormalities identified on H&E stain and other histochemistry will be discussed later in in *Section B* (*Chapter 1 and 2*).

Toluidine stain is considered the stain most routinely used in nerve pathology. Compared to H&E, toluidine stain helps the pathologist to identify the major neuropathic process occurring in the disease whether axonal, demyelinating, or remyelination abnormalities. Other histochemical reactions are also essential in muscle biopsies to reveal the biochemical integrity of fiber types and their selective involvement in the disease process. They also detect the presence or absence of a particular enzyme such as those used in mitochondrial dysfunction.

In excess, histochemistry can also demonstrate the structural changes in the muscle that are apparently visualized on routine histological stains. The major histochemical reactions used in neuromuscular pathology are summarized in Table 7.1.

Each muscle stain (general, special, or oxidative reaction) has its own protocol. This protocol describes the concise technical steps every technologist must follow to prepare these stains.

7.2 Histochemistry Protocol

In this section, we list the histochemical protocols that form our routine panel of muscle and/or nerve histochemistry. **Table 7.2** summarizes the materials and the technical steps used in the manual preparation of each histochemical stain and enzymatic reaction. Although each laboratory has its own manual, the standard principles and chemical solutions used in the preparation are usually similar. All histological and histochemical techniques are performed from frozen sections and mounted on positive charged slides. Sections can also be stored frozen until required and should be air dried again before use.

7.3 Immunohistochemistry (IHC)

Immunohistochemistry (IHC) is an additional laboratory tool used in the assessment of muscle tissue pathology. It is complementary to histology and special histochemistry; its findings help the pathologist to reach a diagnosis when differential etiologies are listed. The technique itself evaluates the protein expression in the tissue and does not reflect the gene coding sequence or RNA activity. Therefore, its interpretation should be carefully carried out. The immunolabeling index should be contained in the same final report, rather than described in a separate report.

IHC applies on both sarcolemmal proteins, such as dystrophin, and sarcoplasmic antigen receptors (**Table 7.3**). Several manufactured antibodies are now available in the market for studying diseased muscle. In *Chapter 5, Table 5.2* we listed the commonly used IHC antibodies in muscle pathology practice with their manufacture sources. In this section, **Table 7.3** summarizes the histological interpretation and reactions of the sarcolemmal proteins or antibody stains on muscle tissue (**Figure 7.1**).

Table 7.1 Panel of histochemical reactions routinely used in neuromuscular pathology practice.

Histochemical stain	Fiber type distribution	Histochemical reaction on the tissue
ATPase pH4.2	Type I: Dark, Type II: Light	Type I fibers predominant in deltoid/biceps
ATPase pH9.4	Type I: Light, Type II: Dark	Type II fibers predominant in quadriceps
Gomori trichrome	Type I: Dark, Type II: Light	Nuclei: *blue*; Connective tissue: *green*
NADH-TR	Type I: Dark, Type II: Light	*Blue-green* end products
SDH	Type I: Dark, Type II: Light	*Blue-green* end products
COX	Type I: Dark, Type II: Light	Present: *brown gold*; Absence*: white fibers*
COX-SDH	Type I: Dark, Type II: Light	*Blue fibers* are COX-negative fibers
Phosphorylase*	Type I: Light, Type II: Dark	Present: *purple*; Absence: *white fibers*
Phosphofructokinase	Type I: Light, Type II: Dark	Present: *blue-gray*; Absence: *white fibers*
Oil red	Type I: Dark, Type II: Light	Nuclei: *blue*; Lipid deposits: *red*
PAS	Type I: Light, Type II: Dark	Nuclei: *blue*; Glycogen deposits: *pink*
Congo red	Type I: Dark, Type II: Light	Nuclei: *blue*; Amyloid deposits: *red*
MHCf	Type I: Light, Type II: Dark	Type II fibers predominant in quadriceps
MHCs	Type I: Dark, Type II: Light	Type I fibers predominant in deltoid/biceps
Acid phosphatase	No specific fiber distribution	Nuclei: *green*; Positive activity: *red*
Alkaline phosphatase	No specific fiber distribution	Positive activity: *red-brown*
Esterase*	No specific fiber distribution	Positive activity: *orange-brown*

* Phosphorylase should be interpreted immediately as it may disappear within 12–24 hours after staining. Esterase activity highlights denervated fibers and neuromuscular junction as orange-brown.

Note: Although each stain has its own fiber type distribution, *period acid-Schiff (PAS), phosphorylase, ATPase 9.4,* and *fast-myosin heavy chain* (MHCf) are the only stains that show type I fibers lighter than type II fibers.

Table 7.2 Histochemistry protocols used in our lab to prepare special staining of muscle or nerve.

Histochemical stain	Materials	Protocol
Gomori trichrome (GT) stain	a. Glacial acetic acid b. Harris hematoxylin c. Ammonium hydroxide d. Distilled water e. GT mixture Bluing solution: c+d	1. Cut 10-micron sections through cryostat 2. Immerse sections in hematoxylin ×10 min 3. Rinse it in tap water 4. Immerse it in bluing solution ×30 sec 5. Wash it with water 6. Immerse sections in GT mixture ×10 min 7. Incubate in acetic acid 8. Immerse rack with sections in alcohol 9. Clear with xylene ×5 min 10. Mount coverslip in Permount medium
Periodic acid-Schiff (PAS)	a. Glacial acetic acid b. Chloroform c. Dimedone d. Periodic acid e. Alcohol f. Schiff reagent g. Distilled water Carnoy's solution: a+b+e Dimedone solution: c+e	1. Cut 10-micron sections through cryostat 2. Add slide in Carnoy's solution ×5 min 3. Rinse several times in distilled water 4. Place in periodic acid ×5 min 5. Rinse several times with distilled water 6. Place it in 5% dimedone solution ×15 min 7. Wash it twice with distilled water 8. Immerse it in Schiff reagent ×15 min 9. Run it in the water tap ×5 min 10. Dehydrate in alcohol different concentration 11. Clear with xylene and mount in medium

Table 7.2 Histochemistry protocols used in our lab to prepare special staining of muscle or nerve. (Continued)

Histochemical stain	Materials	Protocol
Oil red stain	a. Harris hematoxylin b. Oil red O c. Propylene glycol d. Formaldehyde 37% e. Sodium phosphate monobasic f. Sodium phosphate dibasic g. Distilled water Phosphate solution: d+e+f+g Oil red solution: b+c	1. Cut 10-micron sections through cryostat 2. Place slide in phosphate solution ×5 min 3. Wash it twice in distilled water 4. Place it twice by propylene glycol ×2 min 5. Place slide in Oil red solution ×30 min 6. Differentiate slides in propylene ×1 min 7. Rinse slides in distilled water 8. Immerse slides in hematoxylin ×2 min 9. Rinse slide thoroughly in tap water 10. Rinse slide twice in distilled water 11. Coverslip with an aqueous mounting
Cytochrome C oxidase (COX)	a. Cytochrome C b. Catalase c. Diaminobenzidine tetra HCL d. Distilled water e. Sodium phosphate monobasic f. Sodium phosphate dibasic *Phosphate solution: d+e+f COX solution: a+b+c+d+*	1. Cut 10-micron sections through cryostat 2. Incubate the slide in COX solution ×1.5 h 3. Rinse it in distilled water 4. Place it in formol-calcium ×10 min 5. Rinse it in tap water 6. Dehydrate it in alcohol 7. Clear it with xylene and mount in medium

(continued)

Table 7.2 Histochemistry protocols used in our lab to prepare special staining of muscle or nerve. (Continued)

Histochemical stain	Materials	Protocol
Succinate dehydrogenase (SDH)	a. Sodium succinate b. Phenazine methosulphate c. Nitrotetrazolium blue chloride d. Potassium cyanide e. Distilled water f. Sodium phosphate monobasic g. Sodium phosphate dibasic *Phosphate solution: f+g SDH solution: a+b+c+*	1. Cut 10-micron sections through cryostat 2. Incubate the slide in SDH solution for 1.5 h 3. Rinse it in distilled water 4. Place it in formol-calcium ×10 min 5. Rinse it in tap water 6. Dehydrate it in alcohol 7. Clear it with xylene and mount in medium
Combined SDH + COX	Both COX and SDH materials and solutions preparation	1. Cut 10-micron sections through cryostat 2. Incubate the slide in COX solution ×1.5 h 3. Leave it in distilled water 4. Incubate the slide in SDH solution ×1 h 5. Rinse it in distilled water 6. Dehydrate it in alcohol 7. Clear it with xylene and mount in medium
Reduced nicotinamide adenine dinucleotide tetrazolium reductase (NADH-TR)	a. β-Nicotinamide A dinucleotide b. Hydrochloric acid c. Nitrotetrazolium blue chloride d. Distilled water e. Tris buffer NADH solution: a+c+e	1. Cut 10-micron sections through cryostat 2. Incubate in NADH solution ×45 min 3. Rinse in distilled water 4. Place in 10% formalin ×10 min 5. Rinse in distilled water 6. Coverslip using a mounting medium

(continued)

Table 7.2 Histochemistry protocols used in our lab to prepare special staining of muscle or nerve. (Continued)

Histochemical stain	Materials	Protocol
Phosphorylase	a. Glacial acetic acid b. Adenosine-5-monophosphate c. Glucose-1-phosphate d. Potassium iodide e. Iodine f. Acetate buffer g. Distilled water h. Ethanol i. Glycogen	1. Cut 10-micron sections through cryostat 2. Incubate in incubation medium ×1 h 3. Immerse it in Lugol's solution 4. Rinse in distilled water 5. Coverslip using a mounting medium
	Lugol's solution: d+e+g Incubation medium: b+c+f+h+i	

Note: Most of the materials mentioned here have already been described before.

Although these antibodies were designed for the use of fixed paraffin sections, the protocols have been adjusted by the manufacturer to work on frozen sections. Therefore, the technologist should select *IHC-F* type during the order from the manufacturer. The IHC stain may not give satisfactory results if it is done on paraffin fixed sections. However, the antibody staining on the frozen unstained slides would give the best results. It is unnecessary to keep the unstained slides permanently in the freezer.

Some of these antibodies are concentrated so the dilution and optimization should be performed before using them in the IHC process in order to maintain standardized quality assurance. The validation requires positive and negative control. The selected antibody should be mouse or rabbit monoclonal and react with human. The technologist should stay informed of the antibody quality via website reviews or through previously published papers using the same antibody.

Assessment of each protein individually in serial sections is necessary to ensure that the antibodies are working. While the technologist adds the positive control on the diagnostic slides, the pathologist should be aware of muscle–protein interaction. This interaction has been described in *Table 1.1, Chapter 1*. For example, dystrophin protein deficiency may be accompanied with deficiency of sarcoglycan and dystroglycan staining.

Table 7.3 Histological interpretation of most commonly used sarcolemmal and sarcoplasmic proteins in muscle pathology practice. (*Check Table 1.1; Chapter 1.*)

Muscle protein	Histological interpretation
Sarcolemmal dystrophin- *all domains*	
Uniformly present	Normal
Absent	Duchenne muscular dystrophy (DMD)
Very weak	DMD or DMD carrier, regenerating fibers
Patchy	Becker muscular dystrophy (BMD) or carrier
Sarcolemmal β-spectrin—*control for dystrophin*	
Uniformly present	Normal
Absent	Necrotic fibers
Reduced	*Immature fibers, regenerating fibers, DMD*
Sarcolemmal sarcoglycan (α, β, γ, δ)	
Uniformly present	Normal
Absent all	Limb-girdle muscular dystrophy (LGMD)
Absent in one	*Query* LGMD
Reduced all	DMD, BMD, LGMD
Sarcolemmal dystroglycan (α, β)	
Uniformly present	Normal
Absent	Congenital muscular dystrophy (CMD)
Reduced all	CMD, DMD
Sarcoplasmic dysferlin	
Uniformly present	Normal
Absent or reduced	LGMD type IIB
Sarcolemmal caveolin-3	
Uniformly present	Normal
Absent	LGMD type 1C, hypercreatin kinesemia— Rippling muscle disease
Reduced	Long QT-syndrome, familial hypertrophic cardiomyopathy
Emerin	
Uniformly present in nuclei	Normal
Absent	Emery–Dreifuss syndrome (EDS)
Sarcolemmal merosin (Laminin-α2**)**	
Uniformly present	Normal
Absent or reduced	Merosin deficiency or Danon disease

Table 7.3 Histological interpretation of most commonly used sarcolemmal and sarcoplasmic proteins in muscle pathology practice. (*Check Table 1.1; Chapter 1.*) (Continued)

Muscle protein	Histological interpretation
Sarcolemmal laminin β1	
Uniformly present	Normal
Absent or reduced	LGMD type 2I, Bethlem myopathy
Sarcolemmal utrophin	
Uniformly present	Normal
Highly expressed	DMD, regenerating fibers
Collagen VI	
Uniformly present	Normal
Absent or reduced	CMD "Ullrich syndrome"
Desmin	
Normal	Faint equal staining
Highly expressed	Regenerating fibers
Aggregation	Myofibrillar myopathy, titinopathy

Note: Be aware that some of these muscle proteins can interact with other proteins in the chain.

Manual preparation of IHC is an outdated procedure. This is common in places where advanced technology is not available. To perform automated IHC tissue processing, the following components should be available in the lab:

- Automated immunostainer such as Ventana system
- Detection system: DAB kit
- Bulk fluid used in the immunostainer
- Commercial antibodies kit

Many commercial antibodies from several companies can work on different automated immunostainers.

Interpretation of results depends on several factors including reviewing the technique used, appropriate controls, and maturity of the muscle and nerve fibers. The staining quality is different between laboratories, even though they use the same antibodies with the same detection kit. Therefore, each laboratory should establish its own optimal and standard protocol and baselines. Positive and negative controls are also essential to check for nonspecific background and to determine the antibody's working status. The

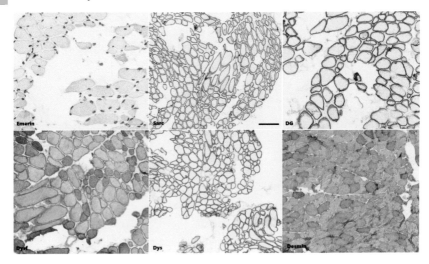

Figure 7.1 Commonly used sarcolemmal and sarcoplasmic muscle proteins. Sarc: sarcoglycan; DG: dystroglycan; Dysf: dysferlin; Dys: dystrophin.

antibody stains, e.g., dystrophin expression, should be analyzed in correlation with clinicopathological findings. If the pathologist believes that the results do not match the clinical and pathological picture or the staining quality is uncertain, the test must be repeated. The result of protein expression usually approximates the diagnosis 80% while the remaining 20% can be left for further tests such as molecular studies.

Figure 7.2 shows a dystrophin labeling on a 31-year-old woman who presented with sudden ventilation-dependent respiratory failure. The pathological picture was not consistent with the clinical picture; however, the dystrophin-2 stain was very weak even when repeated twice. In this case, the pathologist should assess the finding very carefully, and also should confirm that the tissue quality, technical processing, and reagent viability were all satisfactory. The point here is that not every IHC-result gives a meaningful outcome.

7.4 Histological Artifacts

Histological examination can be limited by a number of alterations in tissue sections that occur due to the presence of artifacts. An artifacts is defined as something observed in scientific investigation that is not naturally present, but occurred as a result of an error in the procedure. Histopathological artifacts may occur during surgical removal, fixation, freezing, tissue processing, microtomy, and staining and mounting procedures. It is essential to identify

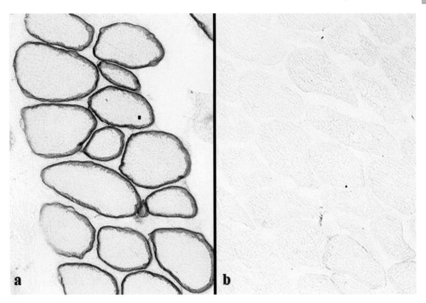

Figure 7.2 Serial sections from a 31-year-old woman with a sudden onset of ventilation-dependent respiratory failure. **(a)** Normal sarcolemmal labeling of dystrophin-2. **(b)** Patient's section shows weak to absent dystrophin-2 protein. This could be either a diagnostic feature of a female carrier of DMD or a primary antibody defect.

the commonly occurring artifacts during histopathological examination of tissue sections. This will help pathologists or technologists to avoid the problem in the future.

It is rare to see artifacts occurring in the prefixation stage. However, if the muscle piece is left at room temperature for a long period of time, autolysis may occur. The autolysis destructs the tissue spaces and may also desaturate DNA, in which case the oxidative enzymes would not function well. The most common artifacts occurring in the muscle tissue fixation stage are **freezing artifacts**. The freezing procedure follows organized steps in which any improper technical mishandling may cause major cellular damage. Freezing artifacts (**Figure 7.3d**) appear as Swiss cheese holes. They represent areas where ice crystals damage the tissue. This mechanism is caused by the osmotic damage derived from ice formation. However, if the samples are kept too moist before freezing, fluid accumulates in the sample and the fibers become disrupted and vacuolated. If there is a long delay before freezing, depletion of glycogen occurs, and this may misdiagnose some suspected metabolic diseases.

49

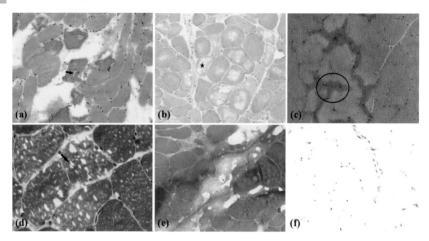

Figure 7.3 Types of histological artifacts. **(a)** Muscle tissue shrinkage and cracks (*black arrow*) due to over drying before freezing. **(b)** Ice crystals artifacts seen as holes (*star*) due to either slow freezing or over warming. **(c)** Stripping appearance of the muscle tissue with hypercontraction due to improper treatment in alcoholic solution or lifting the slides quickly during staining. **(d)** Freezing artifacts (*black arrow*) are due to crystal damage or too much saline. **(e)** Overstaining and hypotonic expression due to either overusage of saline or error in blue buffer formation. **(f)** False negative immunostain expression. ×25.

Allowing the tissue to become dry prior to freezing can also cause muscle fiber shrinkage and cracking (**Figure 7.3a**). This may give false impression of small fibers or improper cracking pathology.

Other common artifacts are **ice-crystal artifacts** that appear as holes in the fibers (**Figure 7.3b**). These artifacts look similar to freezing artifacts but with different mechanism. They are induced by slow freezing of the section allowing the sample to warm up during its transfer from or to the cryostat or freezer. It also results from inappropriate quenching techniques or selection of sections too large for rapid freezing. If the sample is badly affected by freezing artifacts, it can be quickly refrozen. The fibers may become round in shape, but the number of holes is reduced; thus, the overall appearance of the sections improves. Carbon dioxide expansion freezers are also satisfactory for the prevention of ice crystals in fresh tissue.

It is important to distinguish freezing artifacts from the real vacuoles or cores. This can be done by repeating the procedure, looking at different slides, and examining the slides thoroughly.

Rough handling of the sample, improper dehydration by extended time in alcoholic high concentration, or lifting the section off the slide quickly can give a striping appearance as well as fiber hypercontraction. Fibers at the edge of the section become disrupted (**Figure 7.3c**). Extensive saline solution or error in mounting and formation of special stain solution may cause either overstaining or hypotonic expression of the stain (**Figure 7.3e**).

When the tissue sections are flattened in a water bath, air bubbles may become trapped under them. This occurs because of air bubble collapse under the sections, leaving cracked areas after drying. This can be prevented by using freshly boiled water in a flotation bath.

Lastly, immunostaining technical problems may cause false negative protein expression. This may occur due to expired IHC antibody, expired or deficient reagents, or improper protocol application (**Figure 7.3f**). Repeating the stains twice is important to avoid any missing diagnosis.

References

Arikawa E, Ishihara T, Nonaka I, et al. Immunocytochemical analysis of dystrophin in congenital muscular dystrophy. J Neurol Sci. 1991; 105: 79–87.

Bancroft JD, Stevens A. The theory and practice of histological techniques, 3rd edition. Churchill Livingstone, Edinburgh. 1990.

Betz RC, Schoser BG, Kasper D, et al. Mutations in CAV3 cause mechanical hyperirritability of skeletal muscle in rippling muscle disease. Nat Genet. 2001; 28: 218–219.

Brockington M, Brown SC, Lampe A, et al. Prenatal diagnosis of Ullrich congenital muscular dystrophy using haplotype analysis and collagen VI immunocytochemistry. Prenat Diagn. 2004; 24: 440–444.

Clerk A, Morris GE, Dubowitz V. Dystrophin-related protein, utrophin, in normal and dystrophic human foetal skeletal muscle. Histochem J. 1993; 25: 554–561.

Dubowitz V, Pearse AGE. Enzymic activity of normal and diseased human muscle: a histochemical study. J Pathol Bacteriol. 1961; 81: 365–378.

Engel W, Cunningham G. Rapid examination of muscle tissue. Neurology. 1963; 13(11): 919–923.

Fanin M, Angelini C. Muscle pathology in dysferlin deficiency. Neuropath Appl Neurobiol. 2002; 28: 461–470.

Godlewski HG. Are active and inactive phosphorylase histochemically distinguishable? J Histochem Cytochem. 1963; 11: 108–112.

Majer F, Vlaskova H, Krol L, et al. Danon disease: a focus on processing of the novel LAMP2 mutation and comments on the beneficial use of peripheral white blood cells in the diagnosis of LAMP2 deficiency. Gene. 2012; 498: 183–195.

Round JM, Matthews Y, Jones DA. A quick, simple and reliable histochemical method for ATPase in human muscle preparations. Histochem J. 1980; 12: 707–710.

Sabatelli P, Squarzoni S, Petrini S, et al. Oral exfoliative cytology for the non-invasive diagnosis in X-linked Emery–Dreifuss muscular dystrophy patients and carriers. Neuromuscul Disord. 1998; 8: 67–71.

Histochemistry Protocol

Takeuchi T. Histochemical differentiation of phosphorylase a, phosphorylase b and phosphorylase-kinase. J Histochem Cytochem. 1962; 10: 688.

Taqi SA, Sami AA, et al. A review of artifacts in histopathology. J Oral Maxillofac Pathol. 2018; 22(2): 279.

CHAPTER 8

GENETIC BASIS OF NEUROMUSCULAR DISORDERS

Ashraf Dallol, PhD and Maher Kurdi, MD

Contents

Several neuromuscular disorders (NMDs) affecting the muscles and nerves are hereditary or associated with sporadic gene mutations. However, the phenotypes vary from person to person even in the same family. The majority of NMDs have an underlying genetic basis and are inherited in a Mendelian fashion as either autosomal recessive, autosomal dominant, or x-linked. Defects in the mitochondrial genome can also lead to certain types of NMD. In this chapter we will review the genetic basis of NMDs and discuss the different types of genetic tests currently available for use by clinicians.

The Online Mendelian Inheritance in Man (OMIM) database currently lists more than 700 disorders with muscle diseases. Hundreds of genes have already been identified and listed as the main cause of any particular disorder. For example, consider the muscle diseases caused by mutations in the dystrophin (DMD) gene on chromosome xp21.2-21.1. The nature and type of the mutation in the DMD gene are associated with the severity and subtype of DMD causing either Becker muscular dystrophy (BMD) or the more severe Duchenne muscular dystrophy (DMD). Both disorders share the progressive atrophy of muscles leading to cardiomyopathy in adolescence and death in the second decade for DMD or survival beyond this point for BMD.

Genetic testing for NMDs is crucial for several reasons. It can pinpoint the disease in a cost-effective manner while avoiding a lengthy and costly route to diagnosis that often involves invasive muscle or nerve biopsies, magnetic resonance imaging (MRI), electromyography (EMG), and numerous blood tests and profiles. If a gene variation is identified in a patient, then a targeted clinical testing can follow to confirm the diagnosis. An added value for genetic testing is that in the case of familial NMDs, other members of the same family can be tested. This approach will save time and resources and enhance the clinical care of NMD patients. Testing the whole family will confirm that the mutant gene is pathogenic and not variant of unknown significance. Genetic testing will also identify carriers for the disease and help prevention by facilitating premarital testing or preimplantation genetic diagnosis.

Genetic testing is a requirement for indicated companion diagnostics in the case of the new therapies such as the one used in the treatment of DMD.

Genetic testing for NMDs may involve a single-gene targeted approach, multiple-gene approach, or the more inclusive whole-exome or whole-genome sequencing.

8.1 Single or Multiple Gene Approach

In the single-gene approach, the practitioner has a clear idea about the causative gene, either by clinical testing or muscle biopsy findings, and orders a confirmatory test; or as in companion diagnostics, the single-gene test is necessary to determine suitability to receive treatment (e.g., Exondys 51 and DMD). In the multi-gene approach, next generation sequencing (NGS) technology is utilized to perform an expanded and specific analysis of a predetermined panel of genes that are grouped together based on shared phenotype. For example, the practitioner can order gene sequencing using a muscular dystrophy panel or myotonic dystrophy panel. However, if the targeted approach fails to identify the genetic cause of the disease, testing utilizing whole-exome sequencing (WES) or even the more inclusive whole-genome sequencing (WGS) is recommended (**Figure 8.1**).

The single-gene approach typically involves the sequencing, using the chain termination method (CTM), of one gene at a time. Genomic DNA from the patient is prepared from blood, saliva, or buccal swabs. Then the gene of interest is amplified using polymerase chain reaction (PCR) and oligonucleotide primers targeting the regions of interest in the gene, which can be a region acting as a hotspot for mutations or all the coding exons including the splice-site junctions. The sequencing of the amplicons is performed using CTM on dedicated DNA analyzers. This approach is considered the gold standard of DNA sequencing due to the extremely low error rates in the process. However, the sequence output is limited, and it is informative only if a mutation is identified (**Figure 8.1**).

On the other hand, multiplex ligation-dependent probe amplification (MLPA) is another technique widely used for the detection of copy number change, deletions, or duplications in single genes. For example, MLPA could be useful for a screening of patients who could benefit from Exondys 51 and

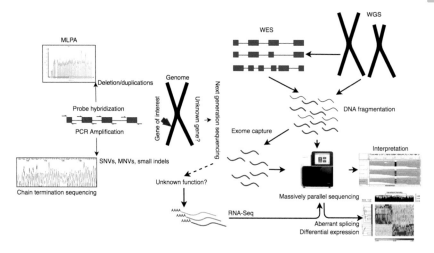

Figure 8.1 Schematic representation of the options available for genetic testing depending on the approach and the phenotype observed.

have an exon 51 skipping in the DMD gene. The MLPA assay is a modified form of multiplex polymerase chain reaction where all targeted exons are hybridized into two specially modified oligonucleotide probes that will bind targets adjacent to each other. This binding is sequence specific and highly sensitive to mismatches. Following successful ligation of the two probes, the amplification of that is detected on DNA analyzers. Because MLPA uses a dedicated reference for every gene, the MLPA targets can be quantified and a deletion or duplication is detected.

The utility of targeted genetic testing is limited when a diagnosis of NMDs cannot be ascertained or suggested from the clinical phenotype. The development of NGS in past decades and the continuous trend of increasing affordability and accuracy allows for the "shot-gun" approach of genetic testing to be utilized even as a front-line test for NMDs.

8.2 Whole-Exome and Whole-Genome Sequencing

WES and WGS are used when the targeted approach fails to identify the genetic cause of the disease. Both tests have a high probability of success in identifying the mutations responsible for an observed phenotype in an NMD patient.

WGS is a technique where the complete human genome is sequenced, and mutations are identified whether they are single nucleotide variants, deletions, or duplications. Furthermore, WGS has the potential to identify trinucleotide repeat expansion, the majority of which are located in non-coding regions and therefore missed in WES. The WES technique is a very useful prelude to WGS as it provides a significant opportunity to identify the pathogenic variant with reduced cost, faster turn-around time, and easier interpretation compared to WGS. The starting material for both WGS and WES is genomic DNA typically extracted from mononucleated cells in the patient's peripheral blood. The genomic DNA is fragmented and processed into barcoded "libraries," which are then sequenced on specialized platforms; the selection of which depends on throughput needs and application (**Table 8.1**).

The sequencing data generated is processed by bioinformatic pipelines aiming to identify and annotate the variants in the sample. A key output is variant classification according to the American College of Medical Genetics and Genomics (ACMG) guidelines: pathogenic, likely pathogenic, variants of unknown significance, likely benign, benign.

One of the arguments against using WGS or WES as front-line diagnostic testing for NMDs is that the data obtained will contain numerous variants of unknown significance or pathogenic variants in genes of unknown function, which may limit the widespread use of such techniques due to the considerable expertise necessary for interpretation and issuing diagnostic reports.

8.3 RNA Sequencing

RNA sequencing (RNA-Seq) of patient samples has recently emerged as a complementary technique with very promising diagnostic yield. It uses the capabilities of high-throughput sequencing methods to provide an insight into cellular transcriptome and total cellular content of RNAs including mRNA, rRNA, and tRNA. It can also tell us which genes are turned on, what are their levels of expression, and at what time they are activated. It specifically facilitates identification of spliced transcripts, post transcriptional modification, gene fusion, mutation/SNP changes, and also finds differences in gene expression between two or more conditions. The latter is called the *differential expression* process.

Initially, the technique was performed through a Sanger sequencing method, which was low-throughput, costly, and inaccurate. Recently, RNA-Seq is performed via NGS technology, which can prepare libraries of RNA instead of DNA; the data is interpreted as changes in the transcriptome of gene expression, aberrant splicing, or globally as alterations in cellular

Table 8.1 Genetic testing approach, techniques used, and platforms with projected data yields.

Approach	Technique	Outcome	Platform	Throughput	Manufacturer
Single gene	CTS MLPA	SNV, MNV, indels Deletion/duplication	3500 G-analyzer	Low	Thermo Fisher
Multigene	NGS	SNV, MNV, indels Deletion/duplication	Miseq NextSeq 550 NovaSeq 6000 S5 system	Low Medium High Medium	Illumina Thermo Fisher
WES	NGS	SNV, MNV, indels Deletion/duplication	NextSeq 550 NovaSeq 6000 S5 system	Low High Low	Illumina Thermo Fisher
WGS	NGS	SNV, MNV, indels Deletion/duplication	NovaSeq 6000	High	Illumina
RNA-Seq	NGS	Aberrant splicing Differential expression	NextSeq 550 NovaSeq 6000 S5 system	Medium High Medium	Illumina Thermo Fisher
Mitoch-DNA sequencing	NGS	SNV, MNV, indels Deletion/duplication	Miseq NextSeq 550 NovaSeq 6000 PGM S5 system	Low Medium High Low Medium	Illumina Thermo Fisher

Abbreviations: CTS: chain termination sequencing; MLPA: multiplex ligated probe amplification; SNV: single nucleotide variant; MNV: multiple nucleotide variant; Indels: insertion-deletion; NGS: next generation sequencing; WES: whole-exome sequencing; WGS: whole-genome sequencing; Mitoch-DNA: mitochondrial DNA.

pathways that can be used to delineate the underlying mutation. The first step in the technique is RNA isolation followed by complementary DNA (cDNA) library preparation, which can vary with the selection of RNA and between NGS platforms.

The RNA is reverse transcribed to cDNA, which then allows the RNA to pass into NGS workflow. Once the library is prepared, adapters are then added to the terminal sides of the fragment. By this, the cDNA library is then analyzed by NGS, producing short sequences corresponding to both ends of the fragment.

When designing RNA-Seq test, the selection of sequencing platform is important and based on clinical goals. Currently, several NGS platforms are commercially available (**Table 8.1**). The NGS platforms can often be classified as either ensemble-based or single-molecule-based. Currently, the Illumina HiSeq platform is the most commonly applied NGS (ensemble-based) for RNA-Seq and has set the standard for NGS sequencing. Single-molecule-based platforms enable single-molecule real-time (SMRT) sequencing but tend to have a high rate of errors in misalignment and loss of reads.

The classical pipeline for RNA-Seq data is generating FASTQ-format files that contain sequencing reads from the NGS platform. However, mapping RNA-Seq reads to the genome is considerably more challenging than mapping DNA sequencing reads because many reads map across splice junctions.

References

Alfano LN, Charleston JS, Connolly AM, et al. Long term treatment with eteplirsen in nonambulatory patients with Duchenne muscular dystrophy. Medicine (Baltimore). 2019; 98. E15858.

Bradley WG, Jones MZ, et al. Becker-type muscular dystrophy. Muscle Nerve. 1987; 1: 111–132.

Fehr A, Gray J, Luong K, et al. Real-time DNA sequencing from single polymerase molecules. Science. 2009; 323: 133–138.

Han Y, Gao S, et al. Advanced applications of RNA sequencing and challenges. Bioinformatics and Biology Insights. 2015; 9: 29–46.

Hoffman, EP, Brown RH, Kunkel LM. Dystrophin: the protein product of the Duchenne muscular dystrophy locus. Cell. 1987; 51: 919–928.

Katz Y, Wang ET, Airoldi EM, Burge CB. Analysis and design of RNA sequencing experiments for identifying isoform regulation. Nat Methods. 2010; 7: 1009–1015.

Kukurba KR, Montgomery SB. RNA sequencing and analysis. Cold Spring Herb Protoc. 2015; 11: 951–969.

Lalic T, Vossen RHAM, Coffa J, et al. Deletion and duplication screening in the DMD gene using MPLA. Eur J Hum Genet. 2005; 13: 1231–1234.

Rentas S, Rathi KS, Kaur M, Raman P, Krants ID, et al. Diagnosing Cornelia de Lange syndrome and related neurodevelopmental disorders using RNA sequencing. Gene Med. 2020; 22.

Richards S, Aziz N, Bale S, et al. Standards and guidelines for the interpretation of sequence variants: a joint consensus recommendation of the American College of Medical Genetics and Genomics and the Association for Molecular Pathology. Genet Med. 2015; 17: 405–424.

Sharon D, Tilgner H, Grubert F, Snyder M. A single-molecule long-read survey of the human transcriptome. Nat Biotechnol. 2013; 31: 1009–1014.

NEUROMUSCULAR FINAL REPORT

Contents

The neuromuscular pathology report is the final step in muscle and nerve biopsies. It should include the gross description of the specimen, histochemical procedures, microscopic description of histological findings, and the diagnosis. Before submitting the final report, the pathologist should make sure that the report follows standard quality coding and control. The pathologist should also be certain that the report is concise and productive, and it answers the clinical questions. Unfortunately, some pathologists write differential diagnoses similar to clinician thought. At this stage, the pathology report would be absolutely unsatisfactory.

There are three reasons why a clinician asks for pathology report:

- The clinician needs confirmation of his or her clinical findings.
- The clinician needs more information about his or her diagnosis.
- The clinician is searching for the diagnosis.

If the clinician thinks, but is unsure, that the patient has myopathic or neuropathic features, then a muscle pathology report will be efficient to confirm the findings. On the other hand, if the clinician knows that the patient has a myopathic or neuropathic disease, but the clinician needs more information about the patient's disease nature, then the pathologist should help the clinician to find the diagnosis.

Our records show that only 60% of 200 muscle biopsy reports were conclusive for histopathological findings. Thirty percent of the biopsies confirmed a specific diagnosis while 10% of total muscle biopsies did not reach any finding or diagnosis (**Figure 9.1**). This clearly proves that muscle biopsies may not always answer clinician questions.

Because muscle or nerve biopsy procedure is costly and time-consuming, giving an inefficient report would delay patient management. A brief comment

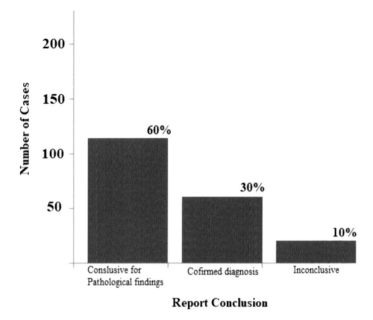

Figure 9.1 An illustrated graph shows the muscle biopsy distribution versus diagnostic conclusion in clinical practice. It is clearly seen that 120 cases (60%) of the biopsies were conclusive while 20 cases (10%) of the biopsies were inconclusive for histopathological findings or diagnosis.

in the report may sometimes stimulate a clinician thought to search for the diagnosis. For example, a 28-year-old woman presented with non-specific muscle symptoms. Clinical investigations were inconclusive for her diagnosis. The clinician asked for muscle biopsy, hoping to find something in the muscle pathology. The biopsy report returned with non-specific findings, but minimal type II atrophic fibers identified. One of the rare differential diagnoses of type II atrophy is myasthenia gravis disease (MGD). The clinician missed ptosis and diplopia during physical examination. After a sequence of other investigations, the case was diagnosed as MGD seronegative for acettylcholine receptor.

There are several templates for muscle biopsy pathology reports. Some pathologists like to mention the histochemistry panel at the beginning of the report and then describe the finding as a story, while others prefer to interpret histological findings with each histochemistry.

The following report style is the formal template used in our neuromuscular lab:

9.1 Muscle Biopsy Report Template

Paraffin embedded sections: H&E stained sections show skeletal muscle in (cross-sectional/longitudinal/both longitudinal and cross-sectional) array. The majority of the muscle fibers maintain polygonal shape and size. There is (minimal/moderate/marked) variation in fiber size. There is (no/yes) evidence of inflammation. Scattered nuclear bag fibers are (seen/not seen).

Histochemistry: The frozen sections of the specimen are stained with H&E, modified Gomori trichrome, and for NADH, ATPase (at pH 4.2, 4.6, and 9.4), esterase, Congo red, and individual and combined SDH/COX.

Frozen sections: H&E stained slides show a skeletal muscle in a cross-sectional array. The fascicles are well populated with muscle fibers. There is (minimal/moderate/marked) variation in muscle fiber caliber owing to the presence of (small round/atrophic/hypoplastic/hypertrophic) fibers that are thoroughly mixed in with fibers of (normal or slightly larger than normal caliber). There is (no/yes) evidence of inflammation. Scattered nuclear bags indicative of severe fiber atrophy are (present/not present). No ring or split fibers are identified. Regenerative and degenerative fibers are (occasionally seen/not seen). Fibers with internalized nuclei are (increased (>3%)/not increased in number) throughout the biopsy.

Trichrome stained sections reveal (no/yes) increase in endomysial connective tissue, ragged red fibers, or abnormal inclusions. ATPase preparations at different concentrations demonstrate a normal checkerboard pattern. There is (fiber type grouping/fiber type predominance/selective atrophy) seen. Both NADH and esterase preparations stain (rare acutely angulated fibers overly dark). (No/yes) moth eaten fibers, target fibers, or fibers with increased accumulations of mitochondria are seen on the NADH preparation. The individual and combined SDH-COX preparation shows (no/yes) COX negative fibers.

A Congo red stain shows (no/yes) evidence of amyloid deposition. PAS stain shows (no/yes) abnormal deposition of glycogen in muscle fibers.

Additional staining: The sections are stained immunohistochemically for MHC-class I and MAC. MHC labels endomysial capillaries (with/without), (minimal/marked) sarcolemmal and/or cytoplasmic staining. There is endomysial capillary (expression/upregulation). It also shows (frequent non-necrotic fibers with cytoplasmic reactivity/cytoplasmic staining in muscle fibers at the periphery of fascicles).

MAC stain shows (no/minimal/marked) expression in myofibers or vasculature. It shows scattered fibers with (sarcolemmal/cytoplasmic) reactivity and (minimal/marked) upregulation in the capillaries (with/without) cytoplasmic staining in focal necrotic fibers.

Oil Red-O stain shows (no/yes) excessive intracytoplasmic lipid deposition in muscle fibers. Myophospharylase activity is (present/absent/reduced).

The sarcolemmal immunolabeling pattern for Dystrophin (*rod domain, C-terminus, N-terminus*) sarcoglycan (α, β, γ, δ), Dystroglycan (α, β), Dysferlin, Spectrin, Merosin, Caveolin-3, Collagen-VI, and Utrophin is (normal/absent).

The appropriate controls are performed and analyzed.

Ultrastructural examination: using electron microscopy is reviewed…

Diagnosis:

Skeletal Muscle. Left/Right-Quadriceps/deltoid, Biopsy: *Diagnosis*

Comment: ……

9.2 Nerve Biopsy Report Template

Paraffin-embedded section is examined. There is (no/yes) evidence of inflammation or amyloid deposition in the formalin-fixed material.

The Epon-embedded material contains a transversely and slightly obliquely orientated multifascicular nerve with (no/minimal) artifactual distortion of the nerve fascicles. There are (no/yes) significant epineural or perineural changes. In particular, there is (no/yes) evidence of inflammation.

There is (no/mild/moderate/marked) degree of loss of myelinated fibers equally from the various fascicles. Otherwise there is a substantial population of large and small myelinated fibers. Many of the former (have/does not have) thinly myelinated sheaths. Unmyelinated large caliber of axons and myelin debris are (not/yes) apparent.

Diagnosis

Nerve, Right/Left-Sural, biopsy: *Diagnosis*

Comment: ….

PART II
MUSCLE

CHAPTER 10

INITIAL APPROACH IN MUSCLE BIOPSY

Contents

Examining a muscle biopsy section under light microscope requires enough experience to interpret the histopathological findings in the proper manner. *The eyes always don't see when the mind doesn't know.*

Because histological changes may sometimes be unequivocal or subtler, pathologists need an organized, systematic approach to evaluate abnormal findings seen in biopsies. Pathologists should not simply tell the clinician whether or not myopathic or neuropathic change exists; they also should help the clinician reach the most probable diagnosis. Indeed, relating the pathology to the clinical picture is paramount to diagnosis.

Once the myopathology is defined, the clinical information is essential for the diagnostic correlation. You may reach the diagnosis by looking only at a hematoxylin and eosin (H&E) section, but most of the time additional sections or stains are required. Knowledge of muscle diseases and their morphological features will definitely make the diagnosis more reachable. In this chapter, we will discuss the initial step in muscle biopsy interpretation, and provide illustrations of the most common pathological findings.

Before looking at the muscle section, make sure that the tissue fragments are adequate, well-stained, and not associated with artifacts. Artifacts can sometimes misdiagnose the case. Common artifacts are summarized in *Chapter 7.*

Bear in mind, not every muscle tissue is abnormal. Abnormal findings in muscle biopsy are usually easily visualized. Upon careful inspection of the tissue section, a pathologist should recognize if the muscle biopsy is normal or abnormal (**Figure 10.1**). If minimal variation in muscle fiber shape and size exists, the pathologist should not call the biopsy abnormal, and additional comments should be provided at the end of the report. The presence of

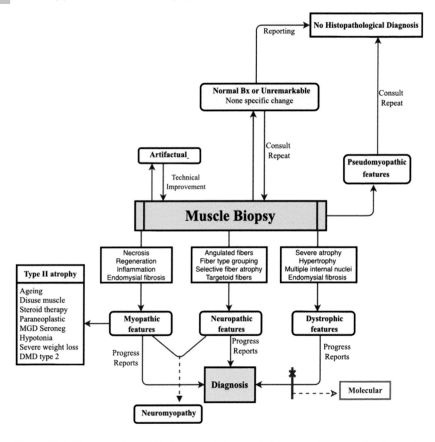

Figure 10.1 Diagram shows initial approach to muscle biopsy. *MGD: myasthenia gravis disease; DMD: Duchenne muscular dystrophy.*

minimal variability in muscle fibers can be seen in patients who are elderly and those with general chronic diseases.

Three major parameters that the pathologist should evaluate in muscle biopsy include: (1) variability in muscle fiber shape and size; (2) focal muscle changes; and (3) presence of inflammation. The best initial approach to differentiate abnormal muscle biopsy is to categorize them as either myopathy, neuropathy, or dystrophy (**Table 10.1**). This method is commonly used by most specialized muscle pathologists during biopsy interpretation.

Some histological features should not mimic abnormal findings. For example, selective type II hypertrophy is associated with heavily exercised muscles, while selective type II atrophy is seen in disused muscles. Type II atrophy can also be seen in other neuromuscular conditions such as steroid-dependent

Table 10.1 Main histopathological classification of abnormal muscle biopsy.

Neuropathy	Myopathy	Dystrophy
Type I and II fiber atrophy	More type II fibers atrophy	More type I fibers atrophy
Type I fiber hypertrophy	Type I fiber predominance	Increased internal nuclei
More type I fiber predominance	Necrotic fibers	Hypertrophic fibers
Loss of checkerboard pattern	Regenerated fibers	Hypercontracted fibers
Fiber type grouping	Perifascicular atrophy	Necrotic fibers
Small or large group atrophy	Inflammation	Splitting fibers
Small angulated fibers	Endomysial fibrosis	Marked endomysial fibrosis
Targetoid or target fibers	Ring fibers	Moth-eaten fibers
Fibers with cores or whorling		

therapy (**Figure 10.1**). The presence of single or multiple necrotizing muscle fibers may help to rule out any pure neuropathic diseases. Neuropathic process is rarely associated with degeneration or necrosis. A new term in the literature, *neuromyopathy*, describes concurrent features of neuropathic and myopathic change and will be discussed in detail in *Chapter 14*.

10.1 Myopathic Features

The essential histological features that define a biopsy as myopathic are myonecrosis and degeneration. Necrotic muscle fibers are described as severely degenerating or dying muscle fibers that are phagocytosed by macrophages (**Figure 10.2a**). They can also be seen as a pale fiber with no nucleus. Isolated necrotic muscle fibers are commonly seen in metabolic myopathies while clusters of necrotic fibers are seen in inflammatory myopathies or myopathic dystrophy.

Every muscle necrosis is usually accompanied with muscle fiber regeneration. Regenerating muscle fiber is described as a blue-shaped fiber with multiple peripheral nuclei (**Figure 10.2a**). Both atrophic and hypertrophic fibers are not considered indicators for myopathic change. They can both present, either individually or combined, in any muscle disease. Occasionally, type II fiber atrophy is associated more with myopathic diseases such as paraneoplastic-induced myopathy (**Figure 10.1**).

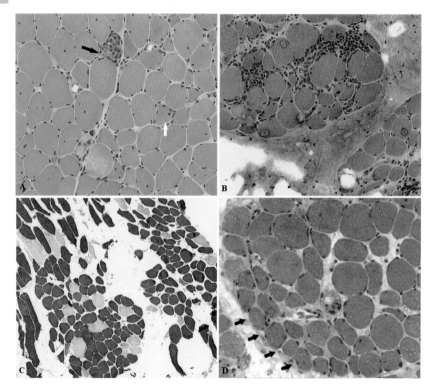

Figure 10.2 Myopathic features. **(a)** H&E section of necrotizing myopathy with phagocytosed necrotic fiber (*black arrow*) and regenerated muscle fiber (*white arrow*). **(b)** Myopathy with endomysial inflammation. **(c)** *Slow* myosin heavy chain shows type I fiber predominance. **(d)** Myopathy with perifascicular atrophy (*black arrows*). Reprinted with permission from Dr. Robert Hammond, Western University, Canada. All images are ×20.

Other abnormal general changes that help to diagnose myopathy are type II fiber predominance, inflammation, ring fibers, and perifascicular atrophy (**Figure 10.2b–d**). If more than 3% of muscle fibers contain centrally positioned nuclei, it suggests myopathic disease.

Specific types of myofibrillar change can diagnose specific types of myopathy, such as tubular aggregates, cytoplasmic bodies, protein aggregates, and central cores. (See *Chapter 11*.)

10.2 Neuropathic Features

Neuropathic process affecting muscles is always a diagnostic challenge. Some pathologists misdiagnose neuropathic features with dystrophy, especially when the features present with only marked hypertrophic and atrophic changes. In fact, a few dystrophic diseases may coexist with neurogenic change such as *facioscapulohumeral dystrophy.*

The clinician must carefully inspect the case in order to distinguish the neuropathic change from dystrophic change. The main histological feature to say this biopsy contains early neuropathic change is the loss of checkerboard pattern accompanied with scattered small dark angulated fibers of type I fibers more than type II fibers (**Figure 10.3c**). Predominant angulated type II atrophy is not a feature of neuropathy and it has several differential diagnoses (**Figure 10.1**). Hypertrophic fibers and fiber-type grouping are considered pathognomonic features of muscle denervation (**Figure 10.2a–b**). They result from collateral sprouting of the nerves that reinnervate the denervated fibers. If the fiber-type is surrounded by fibers of the same type, it is usually considered as a group. Selective grouping of fiber atrophy is another example of the reinnervation process. It is important to distinguish fiber-type predominance from fiber-type grouping. The permanent reinnervation process triggers target/targetoid fiber formation (**Figure 10.3d**). Target fiber is defined as a central rim surrounded by a pale zone within the fiber, indicating an end nerve innervation. This sometimes mimics central core appearance, which makes it difficult to distinguish from targetoid fibers or moth-eaten fibers.

10.3 Dystrophic Features

Dystrophy is a type of myopathic feature but with structural defect in any sarcolemmal protein. It is due to partial degeneration with compensation on different types of muscle fibers. That is the reason why we see hypertrophic and atrophic fibers embedded in a fibrotic background in dystrophy cases (**Figure 10.4**). Because of the perimysial and endomysial fibrosis, the spaces between muscle fibers become widened. Moreover, multiple splitting fibers and internal nuclei are easily seen. A few necrotic fibers can also be found.

Careful clinicopathological correlation is required to histologically differentiate dystrophy from neuropathy in muscle biopsy. Neuropathy is usually not accompanied by multiple internal nuclei, endomysial fibrosis, or necrotic changes. Target/targetoid fibers have never been features of dystrophic disease.

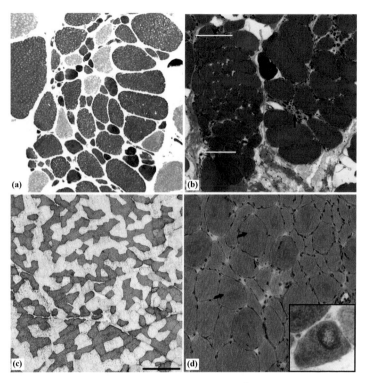

Figure 10.3 Neuropathic features. **(a)** ATPase 4.2 shows fiber-type grouping. **(b)** H&E section with selective group of fiber type atrophy (*between the black arrows and white lines*). **(c)** *Slow*-myosin heavy chain shows small dark angulated muscle fibers. **(d)** H&E stain, with NADH stain on the *small box*, shows target fibers (*black arrows*). *Reprinted with permission from Dr. Robert Hammond, Western University, Canada.*

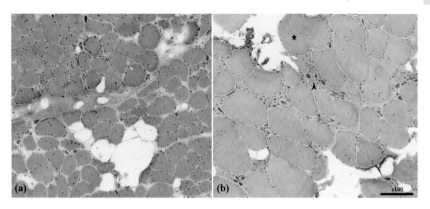

Figure 10.4 (a, b) Dystrophic features. These are hypertrophic fibers (*****) and focal selective atrophic fibers (*black arrow*). ×100.

References

Bilbao JM, Schmidt R, Hawkins C. Diseases of peripheral nerve. In: Love S, Louis DN, Ellison DW (eds) Greenfield's neuropathology, 8th edition. Hodder Arnold, London. 2008; pp. 1609–1724.

Dastur DK, Razzak ZA. Possible neurogenic factor in muscular dystrophy: its similarity to denervation atrophy. J Neurol Neurosurg Psychiatry. 1973; 36(3): 399–410.

Fenichel GM, Emery ES, Hunt P. Neurogenic atrophy stimulating facioscapulohumeral dystrophy. A dominant form. Arch Neurol. 1967; 17(3): 257–260.

Joyce NC, Oskarsson B, Jin Lee-way. Muscle biopsy evaluation in neuromuscular disorders. Phys Med Rehabil Cli N Am. 2012; 23(3): 609–631.

CHAPTER 11
DIFFERENTIAL DIAGNOSIS

Abnormal cytological features in any muscle biopsy are considered essential parameters in the diagnostic approach (Table 11.1) (Figure 11.1). Specific cytoplasmic changes can minimize differential diagnosis into a shorter list. However, additional stains are sometimes required to classify some neuromuscular diseases. The pathologist should combine all these features in the context of clinical information to reach the most probable diagnosis.

Abnormal cytoplasmic changes in muscle biopsy can be categorized into two types:

- Changes affecting the linearization of mitochondria such as ragged red fibers, structural or nonstructural cores, target fibers, and lobulated fibers (Figure 11.1a, b, e). These changes always require additional stains to highlight them. The best markers are oxidative enzymes. For example, ragged red fibers are seen as subsarcoplasmic basophilia in H&E, ragged red fibers in Gomori trichrome, and ragged blue fibers in NADH stain (Figure 11.1a).
- Changes affecting sarcoplasmic proteins and myofibrillar arrays, such as vacuolation and protein aggregates. These changes are explored by using specific histochemical stains and their findings help in the differential diagnosis of some neuromuscular diseases. For example, nemaline rods are rarely seen by H&E thus their appearance requires additional stains. Toluidine stain on plastic section highlights the rods as blue-green (Figure 11.1i).

On the other hand, some protein aggregates may need immunohistochemistry. For example, protein aggregates in myofibrillar myopathy or titinopathy can be stained with desmin.

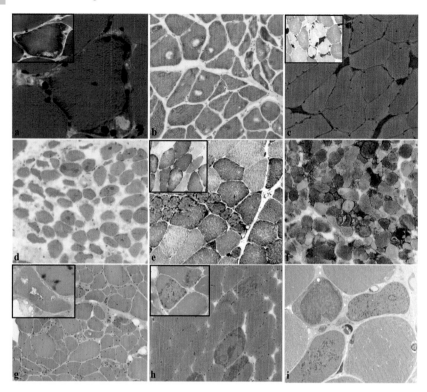

Figure 11.1 Common histopathological features seen in abnormal muscle biopsy. **(a)** Ragged red fiber; H&E section and GT (*small square*). **(b)** Central cores. **(c)** Tubular aggregate; H&E section and NADH (*small square*). **(d)** Cytoplasmic bodies. **(e)** Lobulated trabecular fibers with moth-eaten shape; SDH section and COX (*small square*). *This figure was published in Muscle biopsy: A practical approach, Chapter 4, V. Dubowitz, Histological and histochemical changes, Page 85, Copyright Elsevier 2013.* **(f)** PAS-stained section shows glycogen deposition. **(g)** Rimmed vacuoles; H&E section and GT (*small square*). **(h)** Protein aggregates; H&E section and GT (*small square*). **(i)** Toluidine plastic section shows nemaline rods. *Reprinted with permission from Dr. Robert Hammond, Western University, Canada.*

In **Table 11.1**, we describe the common histopathological features seen in abnormal muscle biopsy with their histochemical findings and differential diagnosis.

Table 11.1 Definitions, histochemical features, and differential diagnoses of abnormal cytological features commonly found in neuromuscular diseases.

Morphological structure	Definition	Histochemical finding	Differential diagnosis
Ragged red fiber	Subsarcolemmal aggregation of mitochondria (**Figure 11.1a**)	**H&E:** subsarcolemmal basophilia **GT:** ragged red fibers **NADH:** ragged blue fibers **COX:** COX-negative fibers **EM:** mitochondrial aggregation, swollen mitochondria, and paracrystallin inclusions	Aging process Mitochondrial myopathy Inclusion body myositis Oculopharyngeal muscular dystrophy Zidovudine therapy Amyotrophic lateral sclerosis Myofibrillary myopathies Myotonic dystrophy (rare)
Central core	Cytoplasmic space in the center of muscle fibers devoid of mitochondria. It is either structural type (retain myofibrillar pattern) or nonstructural type **Figure 11.1b.**	**H&E:** central clearing or eosinophilia **GT:** central clearing **Oxidative enzymes:** central clearing **Desmin:** central aggregation **EM:** fibers devoid of mitochondrial, myofibrillar disruption	Central core myopathy Minicore myopathy Nemaline rod myopathy Titinopathy Filamin C-myopathy Hypothyroid myopathy (rare) Denervation

(Continued)

Table 11.1 Definitions, histochemical features, and differential diagnoses of abnormal cytological features commonly found in neuromuscular diseases. *(Continued)*

Tubular aggregate	Irregular cytoplasmic accumulation containing slits or cracks and found in the periphery of muscle fibers (type II>type I) (**Figure 11.1c**)	**H&E:** peripheral irregular basophilia **GT**: red-green with cracks **NADH:** dark blue **COX/SDH:** negative **PAS:** purple **EM:** hexagonal tubules arranged in honeycombs appearance	Exercised myalgia Tubular aggregate myopathy Hyperkalemic periodic paralysis Myoadenylate deaminase disease Glycogen storage disease "type X" Limb-girdle myasthenic syndrome Stormorken syndrome (rare)
Cytoplasmic body	Small spherical cytoplasmic aggregates in the center of muscle fibers (**Figure 11.1d**)	**H&E:** spherical eosinophilic bodies **GT/NADH:** red **PAS**: blue-purple **EM**: spheroidal bodies with Z-desk aggregation	Inclusion body myositis Collagen vascular disease Myofibrillar myopathy Limb-girdle muscular dystrophy Oculopharyngeal muscular dystrophy Cytoplasmic body myopathy HIV myopathy

Table 11.1 Definitions, histochemical features, and differential diagnoses of abnormal cytological features commonly found in neuromuscular diseases. (Continued)

Rimmed vacuoles	Irregular empty inclusions surrounded by basophilic granules (**Figure 11.1g**)	**H&E:** slits surrounded by blue granules **GT:** red-blue inclusion **TDP-43:** positive inclusion **EM:** osmophilic cytoplasmic debris	Inclusion body myositis Myofibrillar myopathy LGMD type 1a/2g/1F Oculopharyngeal muscular dystrophy Welander distal myopathy Emery-Dreifuss dystrophy (rare) Nonaka myopathy (DMRV)
Lobulated fibers Trabecular fibers Moth-eaten fibers	Peripheral linearization of mitochondria in a triangular shape with central clearing (**Figure 11.1e**)	**H&E:** triangular central clearing **GT:** red **COX/SDH:** dark blue irregularity	Congenital muscular dystrophy Limb-girdle muscular dystrophy 2A Bethlem myopathy Scapuloperoneal muscular dystrophy Steroid myopathy
Nemaline rods	Irregular cytoplasmic spherical rods in the center and periphery of muscle fibers (**Figure 11.1i**)	**H&E:** eosinophilic rods **GT:** green-blue **Toluidine:** light-purple **NADH:** dark-blue **EM:** dense crystalloid bodies	Nemaline rod myopathy Central core myopathy Centronuclear myopathy HIV myopathy Mitochondrial myopathy

(Continued)

Table 11.1 Definitions, histochemical features, and differential diagnoses of abnormal cytological features commonly found in neuromuscular diseases. *(Continued)*

Protein aggregates	Irregular cytoplasmic aggregate of myofibrillar proteins in the muscle fibers or in the vacuoles (**Figure 11.1f, h**)	**H&E:** red-eosinophilic aggregate **GT**: dark blue-red **NADH**: dark blue **PAS**: pink-red (glycogen) **Oil red**: red (lipids) **Desmin**: brown aggregation **EM**: granulotubular filamentous materials	Myofibrillar myopathies Inclusion body myopathies Titinopathy Actinopathies Myosinopathy Glycogen storage disease Lipid storage disease Reducing body myopathy (FHL1)

Abbreviations: EM: electron microscopy; HIV: human immunodeficiency virus; DMRV: distal myopathy with rimmed vacuoles; GT: Gomori trichrome; SDH: succinate dehydrogenase; COX: cytochrome C oxidase; PAS: periodic acid-Schiff; TDP-43: TAR DNA binding protein.

Note: With correlation to Figure 11.1, these features help in the diagnostic approach.

References

Belaya K, Finlayson S, Slater CR, et al. Mutations in DPAGT1 cause a limb-girdle congenital myasthenic syndrome with tubular aggregates. Am J Hum Genet. 2012; 91: 193–201.

Borsani O, Piga D, Costa S, et al. Stormorken syndrome caused by a p.R304W STIM1 mutation: the first Italian patient and a review of the literature. Front Neurol. 2018; 9: 859.

Guerard MJ, Sewry CA, Dubowitz V. Lobulated fibers in neuromuscular diseases. J Neurol Sci. 1985; 69: 345–356.

Hirano M, Angellini C, Montagna P, et al. Amyotrophic lateral sclerosis with ragged red fibers. Arch Neurol. 2008; 65(3): 403–406.

Isaacs H, Heffron JJ, Badenhorst M. Central core disease. A correlated genetic, histochemical, ultramicroscopic, and biochemical study. J Neurol Neurosurg Psychiatry. 1975; 38: 1177–1186.

Keira Y, Noguchi S, Kurokawa R, et al. Characterization of lobulated fibers in limb girdle muscular dystrophy type 2A by gene expression profiling. Neurosci Res. 2007; 57(4): 513–521.

Modi G. Cores in hypothyroid myopathy: a clinical, histological, and immunohistochemistry study. J Neurol Sci. 2000; 175(1): 28–32.

Oates EC, Jones KJ, Donkervoort S, et al. Congenital titinopathy: comprehensive characterization and pathogenic insights. Ann Neurol. 2018; 83(6): 1105–1124.

Ono S, Kurisaki H, et al. Ragged red fibers in myotonic dystrophy. J Neurol Sci. 1986; 74(2–3): 247–255.

Osborn M, Goebel HH. The cytoplasmic bodies in a congenital myopathy can be stained with antibodies to desmin, the muscle-specific intermediate filament protein. Acta Neuropathol. 1983; 62: 149–152.

Rifai Z, Welle S, Kamp C, Thornton CA. Ragged red fibers in normal aging and inflammatory myopathy. Ann Neurol. 1995; 37(1): 24–29.

Schessl J, Feldkirchner S, Kubny C, Schoser B. Reducing body myopathy and other FHL1-related muscular disorders. Semin Pediatr Neurol. 2011; 18(4): 257–263.

Schiaffino S. Tubular aggregates in skeletal muscle: just a special type of protein aggregates. Neuromuscul Disord. 2012; 22: 199–207.

Sharma MC, Goebel HH. Protein aggregate myopathies. Neurol India. 2005; 53(3): 273–279.

Uyama E, Uchino M, Chateau D, et al. Autosomal recessive oculopharyngodistal myopathy in light of distal myopathy with rimmed vacuoles and oculopharyngeal muscular dystrophy. Neuromuscul Disord. 1998; 8: 119–125.

CHAPTER 12
ELECTRON MICROSCOPY

Some pathological abnormalities in skeletal muscle biopsy require electron microscopy (EM) to clarify their structural composition. This is called *ultrastructural change*. To prepare the sections for this level, the EM machine needs to perform a sequence of complicated processes. The technique is costly and requires the expertise of a specialized technologist. To obtain a good quality of muscle sections, the tissue pieces should be kept in 3% glutaraldehyde once received in the lab. Fragments placed in formalin solution may show damaging artifacts and architectural distortion.

In general, EM cannot always be used as a definitive standard measure to confirm the histopathological features that already have been described under light microscope. Its specificity and sensitivity are still low. Nevertheless, other architectural patterns, only visualized by EM, may assist in the diagnosis. For example, tubuloreticular inclusions in cases of dermatomyositis are visualized only ultrastructurally.

EM can also help to confirm some detailed pathological features such as nemaline rods or protein aggregates. Moreover, EM is used as an alternative method when the diagnostician fails to reach a definitive conclusion under regular microscope.

When you look at EM sections, try to identify the most interesting findings rather than spending time interpreting unremarkable changes. If you know that the patient has myopathic features, then you may expect to see ultrastructural change associated with myopathy. This would not add much to the diagnosis. On the other hand, if you know that the patient has myopathy, but you don't actually know what kind of myopathy the patient has, then additional findings will be helpful for the diagnosis. Pathologists should screen sarcoplasm, sarcolemma, and internal nuclear changes for any cytological finding.

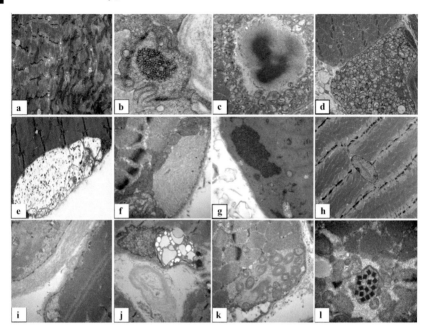

Figure 12.1 Electron microscopy sections show some ultrastructural abnormalities seen in neuromuscular diseases. **(a)** Myofibrillar disruption. **(b)** Tubuloreticular inclusion in endothelial cell. (*Reprinted with permission from Dr. Robert Hammond, Western University, Canada.*) **(c)** Cytoplasmic body. **(d)** Abnormal mitochondrial aggregation. **(e)** Cytoplasmic vacuolations likely rimmed vacuoles. **(f)** Fibrous body. **(g)** Glycogen body. **(h)** Intranuclear filamentous inclusion. **(i)** Amyloid fibrils. **(j)** Autophagic vacuoles. **(k)** Concentric lamellated bodies. **(l)** Paracrystallin inclusions in mitochondria.

The most common abnormality seen in myopathy is myofibrillar disruption (**Figure 12.1a**). This disorganization may affect the Z-line or filamentous bands, based on where it occurs. In necrotic fibers, the myofilament structure is lost and replaced by amorphous granular materials. Other abnormalities may include vacuolation, protein deposition, or abnormalities affecting blood vessels. **Table 12.1** and **Figure 12.1** summarize common ultrastructural abnormalities seen in neuromuscular disorders.

Table 12.1 Some ultrastructural abnormalities seen in muscle diseases and their differential diagnoses.

Ultrastructural abnormality	Differential diagnosis
Tubuloreticular inclusions	Dermatomyositis
Tubulofilamentous inclusions	Inclusion body myositis
	Oculopharyngeal muscular dystrophy
	Emery-Dreifuss disease
	Welander distal myopathy
Paracrystallin inclusions	Mitochondrial myopathy
Curvilinear bodies	Hydroxychloroquine-induced myopathy
Fingerprint bodies	Inflammatory myopathy
	Oculopharyngeal muscular dystrophy
	Fingerprint body myopathy
	Myotonic dystrophy
Autophagic vacuoles	Metabolic myopathy
	Myofibrillar myopathies
	Facioscapulohumeral muscular dystrophy
	Limb-girdle muscular dystrophy
	Amyloidosis
Amyloid fibrils	Amyloidosis
	Hydroxychloroquine-induced myopathy
	Inclusion body myositis
Membrane-bound glycogen	Glycogen storage disease (Pompe disease)
Cytoplasmic bodies	See Table 11.1 in Chapter 11
Nemaline rods	See Table 11.1 in Chapter 11
Tubular aggregates	See Table 11.1 in Chapter 11
Rimmed vacuoles	See Table 11.1 in Chapter 11

CHAPTER 13

CLASSIFICATION OF MYOPATHY

The word *myopathy* is taken from a Greek name (Myo: *muscle* + Pathy: *suffering*), meaning muscle diseases. It clinically implies muscle weakness. Myopathy can be sporadic and hereditary due to genetic mutations or acquired resulting from several systemic diseases. Patients seek medical advice when their symptoms and signs become progressive and unusual.

Weakness is the most reliable clinical indicator of myopathy. Its distribution and progression are variable based on the underlying cause. The clinician categorizes the weakness as proximal type, distal type, or both. Other associated symptoms or signs, given by the patient or detected during the physical examination, can minimize the differential diagnoses. The clinician orders investigations to evaluate a patient's weakness. The most useful blood test used early in the diagnosis is serum creatinine kinase (CK) level. It can be elevated in patients with muscle disorders but may be normal in cases with mild or slowly progressive diseases or patients in end-stage myopathy. CK-MM and CK-MB elevation are typically found in myopathic patients but cannot be used as evidence of associated cardiomyopathy. Some patients with active motor neuron diseases may also have a slightly elevated CK level. So, its serum elevation cannot be used to measure the disease severity.

Electromyography (EMG) is the best clinical investigation tool to diagnose myopathy. (See *Part I, Chapter 3*.) EMG can assist in the classification of myopathies, selection of the biopsy site, and also assessment of the treatment response. A nerve conduction test (NCT) can also be used inferior to EMG to exclude other abnormal neuromuscular conditions. It is typically normal in pure myopathic diseases and abnormal in most neuropathic diseases.

Advances in molecular analysis led to the identification of several gene mutations associated with different types of myopathies. This brought a wider

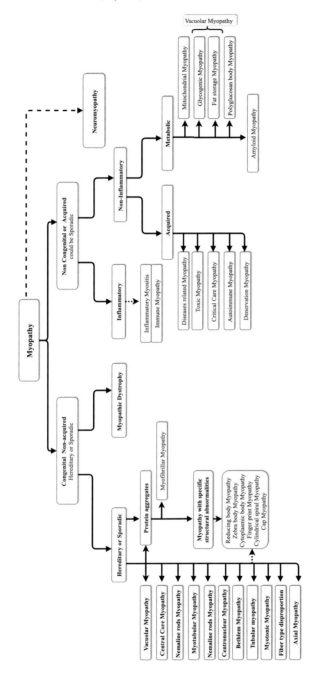

Figure 13.1 Clinicopathological classification of myopathies.

appreciation of their clinical phenotypes. Some forms of myopathic disease are now relatively separate disorders because of their specific gene mutations and morphological features.

Based on all the information mentioned earlier, myopathy is better classified clinicopathologically. For example, when you have a case presenting with myopathic features, you start looking at the cytological details of muscle fibers. Presence of vacuolations means that we deal with "vacuolar myopathy" whereas presence of protein aggregates means we are dealing with "protein aggregate myopathies," such as myofibrillar myopathies (MFM). Both protein aggregates and vacuolations could meet in one clinical diagnosis, MFM. In those cases, we understand that the pathological term *vacuolar myopathy* has been used to describe the clinical diagnosis of MFM. **Figure 13.1** illustrates the clinicopathological classification of myopathies in muscle biopsy practice.

Our approach is to classify myopathy into congenital and acquired forms. The congenital form is usually associated with hereditary or sporadic gene mutations. The acquired form is either due to systemic diseases or could be acquired through sporadic cause. Myopathic dystrophies are categorized under hereditary form as their abnormal genes usually run in the family, such as Duchenne muscular dystrophy (DMD) and Limb-girdle muscular dystrophy (LGMD). Other variants of hereditary or sporadic myopathies may be associated with either specific structural abnormalities or presented with unique histopathological feature. For example, myotubular myopathy (MTM) is characterized by the presence of central large nuclei in every muscle fiber. This disease is hereditary and associated with progressive muscle symptoms.

On the other hand, acquired myopathies due to systemic disease are somewhat difficult to diagnose because of the overlapping clinical features among the chronic disease. Inflammatory myopathies (IM) are immune-mediated acquired myopathies associated with several environmental factors. We cannot classify inflammatory myopathy as hereditary or sporadic disease. For example, inclusion body myositis is commonly associated with mitochondrial mutation, but we cannot say this mutation caused the inflammation.

In summary, the classification of myopathy is different from author to author and from book to book. Our classification system merges the clinical aspect of the diseases with the myopathological features.

References

De Bleecker J. How to approach the patient with muscular symptoms in the general neurological practice?. Acta Neurol Belg. 2005; 105, 18–22.

Werneck LC, Lima JG. Muscle biopsy correlated with electromyography: study of 100 cases. Arch Neuropsiquiatr. 1998; 46: 156–165.

CHAPTER 14

APPROACH TO NEUROMYOPATHY

Contents

The term *neuromyopathy* (*neuropathy* + *myopathy*) refers to a group of neuromuscular diseases associated with concurrent features of neuropathic and myopathic changes in electromyographic (EMG) studies and muscle biopsy. Patients may present with progressive muscle weakness and neuropathic symptoms with or without systemic features. Physical examination and EMG findings can confirm the neuromyopathic nature of this presentation. Histopathological examination through muscle biopsy is strongly indicated as it can show myopathic features (necrotic muscle fibers, regeneration, and atrophy) coexisting with neuropathic features (angulated fibers, fiber-type grouping, and target fibers) (**Figure 14.1**). Bear in mind that a predominant myopathic change with minimal neuropathic background may, but not always, indicate neuromyopathy.

Because of the clinicopathological difficulties in the diagnosis of patients presenting with this rare entity, we created an algorithm approach using microscopic pathology to make the diagnosis for pathologists easier (**Figure 14.2**).

Neuromyopathy can be classified into inflammatory and non-inflammatory subtypes with or without the presence of rimmed vacuoles and protein aggregates. Some literature uses the term *neuromyositis* to refer to neuromyopathy with inflammation. As we described in *Chapter 11, Table 11.1*, protein aggregates are defined as abnormal accumulation of myofibrillar skeletal muscle proteins, which can be seen in several neuromuscular disorders. Rimmed vacuoles are scattered vacuolations surrounded by basophilic granules. They are best seen with Gomori trichrome (GT) stain. The presence of these vacuoles shortens the list of differential diagnoses.

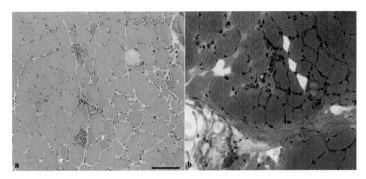

Figure 14.1 Hematoxylin and eosin sections show features of neuromyopathy. **(a)** Myopathic change. **(b)** Neuropathic change with target fibers. ×15.

14.1 Neuromyopathy with Lack of Inflammation

The association of neuromyopathic change and protein aggregates with lack of inflammation, with or without rimmed vacuoles, suggests myofibrillar myopathies (MFM). The presence of neuromyopathic change and rimmed vacuoles with lack of inflammation and protein aggregates expands the differential diagnoses into MFM type V, oculopharyngeal muscular dystrophy (OPMD), Welander distal myopathy (WDM), Emery-Dreifuss dystrophy type II (EDD), distal myopathy with ADSSL1 mutation, Limb-girdle muscular

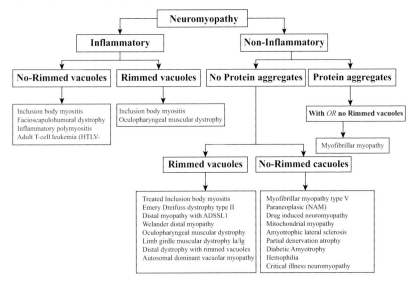

Figure 14.2 A diagram illustrates an algorithm approach to diagnose cases with neuromyopathy.

dystrophy (LGMD) type 1a and 1g, distal dystrophy with rimmed vacuoles (DDRV), and autosomal dominant vacuolar myopathy (ADNM). Treatment history is important in these diseases to rule out healed inflammatory myopathies such as treated inclusion body myositis (IBM). Inflammatory markers (CD4, CD8, and CD68) and major histocompatibility (MHC class-I) expression can enlighten the autoimmune inflammatory process.

Neuromyopathic change with lack of inflammation, lack of protein aggregates, and lack of rimmed vacuoles shorten the differential diagnosis into distal type-MFM, mitochondrial myopathy, paraneoplastic-induced neuromyopathy, drug-induced myopathy, amyotrophic lateral sclerosis (ALS), partial denervation atrophy, and critical care illness.

Chronic hemophilic patients were also found to have neuromyopathic change. Predominant type II atrophy is seen in most of these patients. Diabetic amyotrophy can also present with predominant neuropathic change associated with only minimal myopathic change.

14.1.1 Paraneoplastic-Induced Neuromyopathy

Neurological impairments in patients with malignancies can arise from several factors including chemotherapy, malnutrition, infection, or direct tumor invasion. One of the paraneoplastic complications is neuromyopathy. Subacute sensory and motor neuropathy is commonly associated with small-cell lung cancer but may also occur in other malignancies, including breast cancer, sarcoma, leukemia, and Hodgkin lymphoma. Muscle biopsy findings vary from necrotizing autoimmune myopathy (NAM) associated neuropathic change to predominant type II atrophy, to findings suggestive for nerve vasculitis. CD68-stained macrophages and MHC class-I are always expressed. Rimmed vacuoles and protein aggregate are typically not found in muscle fibers. In few patients, the muscle looks healthy while the inflammation only exists in the perimysium. In this case, further inflammatory markers should be used to identify the type of inflammation.

14.1.2 Drug-Induced Neuromyopathic Change

Drug-induced neuromyopathy is not uncommon in clinical practice. The true frequency of drug-induced complications is difficult to establish because the association cannot always be recognized by the patient or the physician. Drugs causing neuromyopathy include colchicine, lamivudine/telbivudine, amiodarone, hydroxychloroquine, linezolid, and vincristine.

Muscle biopsy histology may show diffuse neuromyopathic changes. Nerve biopsy usually shows axonal degeneration with secondary demyelinating change. Rimmed vacuoles and protein aggregate are typically absent. Electron microscopy (EM) may show mitochondrial change or specific curvilinear bodies, particularly neuromyopathies associated with hydroxychloroquine toxicity.

14.2 Neuromyopathy with Inflammation (Neuromyositis)

The term *inflammatory neuromyopathy* has been described in the literature associated with inclusion body myositis (IBM), facioscapulohumeral muscular dystrophy (FHMD), and LGMD type IIb. The presence of neuromyopathic change with active inflammation and rimmed vacuoles is always associated with IBM. This can be supported by the presence of filamentous inclusions and mitochondrial dysfunction such as ragged red fibers and COX-negative fibers.

OPMD is considered as another differential diagnosis when the patient presents with eye and pharyngeal symptoms, and the biopsy shows dystrophic change.

Severe denervation atrophy can mimic dystrophy. It also can provoke minimal necrotizing myopathy. Target/targetoid fibers seen in denervation with reinnervation resemble fibers with central protein aggregates. However, the only difference between target/targetoid fibers and real protein aggregates seen in other myopathies, such as myofibrillar myopathies, is the associated neuropathic features.

Other rare causes of neuromyositis are systemic lupus erythematosus (SLE), human T-cell lymphotropic virus-type 1 (HTLV-1), and polymyositis. In scleroderma patients, minimal neuropathic features with fibrosis, mild inflammation and myopathic features can also be seen.

CLINICAL CASE

A 50-year-old man presented to the neuromuscular clinic with a 5-year history of progressive weakness of the proximal and distal limbs. He becomes unable to walk without a stander. There is also peripheral tingling sensation, but he denies any double vision, dysphagia, or other unusual systemic symptoms. There is no family history of such presentation.

Neurological examination only demonstrates symmetrical atrophy of the quadriceps muscles and ankle pes cavus. Reflexes are normal. There is no remarkable sensory disturbance.

Serum CK level is elevated (800 IU/L). Other tests, including liver enzymes and serological antibody tests, are unremarkable. EMG study is performed on several muscle groups, which shows minimal myopathic change with positive sharp waves. There is also evidence of mild sensorimotor neuropathy on NCT.

Based on the Above Findings, What is Your Differential Diagnosis?

A biopsy is done from the right deltoid muscle. H&E staining and other histochemistry panels are performed. H&E section, illustrated in **Figure 14.3**, was conclusive.

- Explain the histopathological findings.
- What is your likely diagnosis?

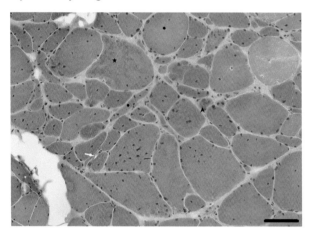

Figure 14.3 H&E section from a 50-year-old man presenting with minimal neuromyopathic features; myopathic changes (*black arrowhead*), neuropathic changes (*black circle*), rimmed vacuole (*white arrow*), cytoplasmic protein aggregate (*).×25.

Interpretation

H&E section shows minimal neuromyopathic features. There are two rimmed vacuoles and scattered cytoplasmic protein aggregates **(Figure 14.3)**. There is no evidence of inflammation. Based on the algorithm approach illustrated in this chapter, the likely diagnosis is myofibrillar myopathy (MFM). Further genetic testing is recommended.

References

Ahmadifard A, Jamshidi J, Tafakhori A, Mollazadeh R, et al. Emery-Dreifuss muscular dystrophy: a report of a large family with 11 affected individuals. Int J Mol Cell Med. 2016; 5(3): 196–198.

Bahri D, Mrabet H, Ben Mrad F, et al. Neuromyositis revealing a systemic lupus erythematosus: a case report. Rev Med Interne. 2004; 25(7): 533–534.

Brais B, Bouchard JP, Tomé FMS, et al. Genetic evidence for the involvement of other genes in modulating the severity of Oculopharyngeal muscular dystrophy (OPMD). Ann Neurol. 1998; 44: 455–456.

Cantarini L, Volpi N, Galeazzi M, Giani T, Fanti F, et al. Colchicine myopathy and neuromyopathy: case report. J Clin Rheumatol. 2010; 16: 229–232.

Defaria CR, De Melo-Souza SE, Pinheiro ED. Hemophilic neuromyopathy. J Neurol Neurosurg Psychiatry. 1979; 42(7): 600–605.

Ferraz AP, Jose FF. Paraneoplastic necrotizing myopathy—a case report. Rev Bras Reumatol Engl Ed. 2017; 57(1): 82–84.

Flanagan EP, Harper CM, St Louis EK, et al. Amiodarone-associated neuromyopathy: a report of four cases. Eur J Neurol. 2012; 19(5): e50–e51.

Goodman B, Boon AJ. Critical illness neuromyopathy. Phys Med Rehabil Clin N Am. 2008; 19(1): 97–110.

Griggs RC, Askanas V, DiMauro S, Engel A, et al. Inclusion body myositis and myopathies. Ann Neurol. 1995; 38: 705–713.

Hermanns B, Molnar M, Schroder JM. Peripheral neuropathy associated with hereditary and sporadic inclusion body myositis: confirmation by electron microscopy and morphometry. J Neurol Sci. 2000; 179: 92–102.

Huser MA, Horrigan SK, Salmikanges P, Torian UM, Viles KD, et al. Myotilin is mutated in limb girdle muscular dystrophy IA. Hum Mol Genet. 2000; 9(14): 214–217.

Koike H, Sobue G. Paraneoplastic neuropathy. Handbook of clinical neurology. 2013; Chapter 41, 115(3). Peripheral nerve disorders.

Kristian B, Anhlberg G, Anvert M, Edstorm L. Welander distal myopathy: an overview. Neuromuscular Dis. 1998; 8(2): 115–118.

Laraki R, Bletry O, Raguin G, et al. 4 new cases of neuromyositis, one of them associated with HTLV-1 infection. Rev Neurol(Paris). 1993; 149(4): 283–288.

Lemmers RJ, Tawil R, Patek LM, Balog J, Block GJ, Santen GW, et al. Digenic inheritance of an SMCHD1 mutation and FSHD-permissive D4Z4 allele causes facioscapulohumeral muscular dystrophy type 2. Nat Genet. 2012; 44: 1370–1374.

Milanov I, Ishpekova B. Differential diagnosis of chronic idiopathy polymyositis and neuromyositis. Electromyogr Clin Neurophysiol. 1998; 38(3): 183–187.

Park HJ, Hong YB, Choi YC, Lee J, Kim EJ, et al. ADSSL1 mutation relevant to autosomal recessive adolescent onset distal myopathy. Ann Neurol. 2016; 2: 231–243.

Selcen D. Myofibrillar myopathies. Neuromuscular Disorders. 2011; 21: 161–171.

Servidei S, Capon F, Spinazzola A, Mirabella M, Semprini S, et al. A distinctive autosomal dominant vacuolar neuromyopathy linked to 19p13. Neurol. 1999; 53: 830–837.

Vieria NM, Naslavsky MS, Licinio L, Kok F, Schlesinger D, et al. A defect in the RNA-processing protein HNRPDL causes limb-girdle muscular dystrophy 1G (LGMD1G). Hum Mol Genet. 2014; 23 (15): 4103–4110.

Xu H, Wang Z, Zheng L, Zhang W, Lv H, et al. Lamivudine/telbivudine-associated neuromyopathy: neurogenic damage, mitochondrial dysfunction and mitochondrial DNA depletion. J Clin Pathol. 2014; 67(11): 999–1005.

Zampollo A, Lisi R, Romagna R. Polymyositis and neuromyositis. Ateneo Parmense 1. 1971; 42(2): 155–164.

CHAPTER 15

APPROACH TO VACUOLAR MYOPATHY

Cytoplasmic vacuoles are a frequent feature in numerous neuromuscular conditions. They are membrane-bound inclusions seen within the muscle fibers, which contain specific cellular components or proteins. They could be non-specific due to the aging process or pathognomonic, based on the whole picture of the case. The terms *vacuolar myopathy* and *autophagic vacuolar myopathy* are commonly used in muscle pathology practice referring to a group of muscle diseases characterized by myopathic features and vacuolations. These vacuoles are always autophagic in nature and vary in their structure and appearance. It is also important to distinguish the vacuoles from freezing artifacts.

It has been scientifically proven that autophagic dysfunction during the cellular catabolic process is considered the main predisposing factor for vacuolar myopathy. This impairment prevents the elimination of misfolded protein aggregates and increases the ability of cellular oxidative stress. As a result, lysosomal breakdown occurs. Several mechanisms in the literature have explained the pathogenesis of these vacuoles (**Figure 15.1**). A selective impairment of cargo sequestration is often encountered in vacuolar myopathies. This may cause a defected chaperone-assisted selective autophagy (CASA) that forms protein-containing vacuoles such as myofibrillar myopathies (MFMs).

Granulophagy defect due to cargo degradation is commonly associated with inclusion body myositis (IBM), and it causes cellular accumulation of stress granules. Moreover, failure of autophagy induction with no formation of autophagosome was detected in some cases of muscular dystrophy as well as

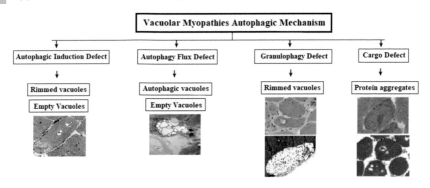

Figure 15.1 Autophagic mechanism in the pathogenesis of vacuolar myopathy.

centronuclear myopathies. An accumulation of undigested cargo also can cause autophagy flux defect, which results in autophagic myopathies (**Figure 15.1**).

Other vacuoles found in some neuromuscular diseases are abnormally formed either due to unclear detected defects or complex autophagic defects. Such diseases include GNE myopathy (distal myopathy with rimmed vacuoles) and some cases of IBM.

Autophagic vacuoles, regardless of their nature, are multilamellated membranous structures found in the sarcoplasm and better illustrated ultrastructurally. In spite of large differences in their etiology and clinical presentation, vacuolar myopathies are grouped together based on their unique histopathology. **Figure 15.2** illustrates a schematic algorithm to diagnose myopathic cases presenting with vacuolation.

The most common vacuolations are rimmed vacuoles (RVs). They are defined histologically as empty inclusions surrounded by basophilic granules. They are commonly seen in IBM, and some other rare neuromuscular diseases such as GNE myopathy, MFM, and autosomal dominant vacuolar myopathy. RVs can be highlighted with Gomori trichrome, P62, TDP-43, or LC3 stains. Some vacuolar myopathies with RVs can also be associated with neuropathic change, which was explained in Chapter 14.

Autophagic vacuolar myopathy (AVM) refers to cases presented with myopathic features and vacuoles containing protein aggregates (**Figures 15.1** and **15.2**). These protein aggregates are seen as eosinophilic solid materials on H&E stain. The most common differential in this list is metabolic myopathy due to glycogen deposition such as Pompe disease. Acid PO4, PAS, and PAS-D are important stains to rule out glycogen storage diseases. However, other causes of autophagic vacuolar myopathies are listed in **Figure 15.2**.

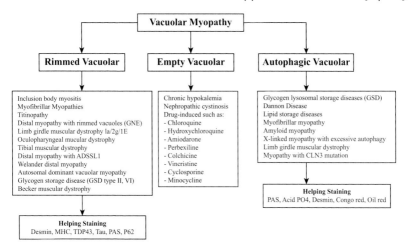

Figure 15.2 Schematic diagram used in the differential diagnosis of vacuolar myopathies in clinicopathological practice.

CLINICAL CASE

A 63-year-old woman presented to the neuromuscular clinic with a 6-month history of proximal muscle weakness of lower limbs and myalgia. The patient is diabetic and suffering from chronic renal insufficiency and chronic liver disease. She is on multiple medications for treatment of diabetes, dyslipidemia, hypertension, and chronic gout.

Neurological examination demonstrates weak quadriceps muscles and normal reflex. There is no remarkable sensory disturbance.

Serum CK level is elevated (1600 IU/L). Her liver enzymes are slightly elevated and serum creatinine level baseline is 221 mmo/L.

EMG study is performed on several muscle groups, which reveals myotonia and spontaneous activity. There is also evidence of mild sensorimotor neuropathy on NCT. Other laboratory investigations including HMGCoR antibody, ANA, and rheumatoid factor are not detected.

Based on the Above Findings, What is Your Differential Diagnosis?

A biopsy is done from her right quadriceps muscle. H&E staining and other histochemistry panels are performed. H&E section is illustrated in **Figure 15.3.**

- Explain the histopathological findings.
- What is your likely diagnosis?

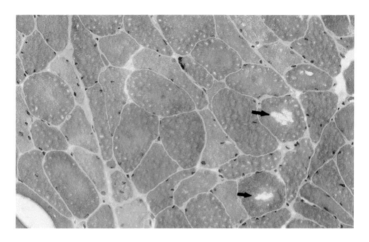

Figure 15.3 H&E section from a 63-year-old woman with colchicine-induced vacuolar myopathy shows muscle fibers with empty vacuoles (*black arrows*).

Interpretation

H&E section shows minimal myopathic change with scattered angulated fibers. There is no inflammation. There are rare empty vacuoles identified in some muscle fibers (**Figure 15.3**). Ultrastructural examination using EM technique does not show any structural defect. After colchicine treatment was withdrawn, patient symptoms improved. The most likely diagnosis of this case is toxic myopathy induced by colchicine treatment.

References

Abdel-Hamid H, Oddis CV, Lacomis D. Severe hydroxychloroquine myopathy. Muscle Nerve. 2008; 38(3): 1206–1210.

Charnas LR, Luciano CA, Dalakas M, et al. Distal vacuolar myopathy in nephropathic cystinosis. Ann Neurol. 1994; 35(2): 181–188.

Dimachkie MM, Baroohn RJ. Inclusion body myositis. Neurol Clin. 2014; 32(3): 629–646.

Le Quintrec JS, Le Quintrec JL. Drug-induced myopathies. Baillieres Clin Rheumatol. 1991; 5(1): 21–38.

Margeta M. Autophagy defects in skeletal myopathies. Ann Review of Path: Mechanism of Diseases. 2019; 15: 261–285.

Radke J, Koll R, Gill E, at al. Autophagic vacuolar myopathy is a common feature of CLN3 disease. Ann Clin Transl Neurol. 2018; 5(11): 1385–1393.

Su F, Miao J, Liu X, Wei X, Yu X. Distal myopathy with rimmed vacuoles: spectrum of GNE mutation in seven Chinese patients. Exp Ther Med. 2018; 16(2): 1505–1512.

Villanova M, Kawal M, Lubke U, Oh SJ, et al. Rimmed vacuoles of inclusion body myositis and oculopharyngeal muscular dystrophy contain amyloid precursor protein and lysosomal markers. Brain Res. 1993; 603(2): 343–347.

CHAPTER 16

MUSCULAR DYSTROPHY DISEASES

Muscular dystrophies (MDs) are a genetically heterogeneous group of degenerative disorders with muscle protein defects characterized by progressive muscle weakness and wasting of variable distribution and severity. Recent advances in molecular genetics have highlighted the diversity of this group of disorders. This spectrum of diseases, comprising several subsets, ranges from severe congenital dystrophies with infantile-onset to milder forms of limb-girdle muscle weakness in adulthood and respiratory compromise. Their classification undergoes constant revision, based on new insights from genetic medicine.

Diagnosis can be established based on characteristic clinical features, distribution of muscle weakness, disease course and age-onset, as well as serum concentration of CK level, muscle histopathology, and genetic findings. In children, the clinical presentation usually starts with delayed walking and poor physical activity in early schooling. Both older children and adults may share similar symptoms such as difficulty rising from a sitting position; difficulty lifting the arms above the head; poor balance; ptosis; and joint contractures. The diseases always progress slowly from muscle weakness and wasting to a wheelchair and complications involving cardiorespiratory functions. The major differential diagnosis is an inflammatory myopathy and congenital muscle weakness.

MDs can be classified clinically into congenital and non-congenital inherited diseases (summarized in **Table 16.1**).

The most common dystrophies are Duchenne muscular dystrophy (DMD) and Becker muscular dystrophy (BMD). Both forms share a defective protein pattern but with variable deficiencies. Many Limb-girdle muscular dystrophies (LGMDs) are autosomal recessive, affecting only one generation

Table 16.1. Muscular dystrophy diseases.

Disease	Pattern	Cause	Clinical features	Investigation	Microscopic Features
Duchenne muscular dystrophy (DMD)	XLR	Dystrophin gene mutation on short arm of Ch.xp21.1-2: • 20% point mutation either frameshift with 40% at exon 55 or missense mutation • 70% deletion/duplication • 5% gonadal mosaic • 5% other new mutations All lead to dystrophin protein deficiency. Female is affected when there is unbalanced translocation of Ch. X. Female becomes carrier.	• Male predominance • Usually late-child onset • Progressive symmetrical proximal limb weakness and wasting • Waddling gait • Gower's maneuver • Calf pseudohypertrophy • Loss ambulation 9–13y • Can be associated with mental retardation, night blindness, cardiomyopathy, or nocturnal hypoventilation	CK is ↑↑ High AST/ALT EMG: myopathy NCT: non-specific **Others to do:** ECG Western blot Gene seq.	• Wide variation in fiber size • Multiple internal nuclei • Hypercontractile fibers • Necrotic and regenerated fibers • Basophilic and rounding fibers • Splitting fibers • Endomysium fibrosis • NADH-TR: moth-eaten fibers • Absent dystrophin stain • Reduced sarcoglycans • Reduced α-dystroglycans • Reduced aquaporin 4 • Overexpressed utrophin • Reduced dystrophin in female
Becker muscular dystrophy (BMD)	XLR	Dystrophin gene mutation on short arm of Ch.xp21.1-2: • 70% point mutation- inframe • 5% mutation in CpG All leads to dystrophin protein deficiency. Worse type: MYF6 <u>Notes:</u> early age, scoliosis, respiratory problems, loss of ambulation by 12y and severe clinical symptoms are seen in DMD>BMD	• Male predominance • Usually late-child onset • Progressive symmetrical proximal limb weakness • Muscle wasting • Calf pseudohypertrophy • Can be associated with mental retardation, joint contracture, and cardiomyopathy	CK is ↑↑ High AST/ALT EMG: myopathy NCT: non-specific **Others to do:** ECG Western blot Gene seq.	• Wide variation in fiber size • Multiple internal nuclei • Hypercontractile fibers • Necrotic and regenerated fibers • Basophilic and rounded fibers • Splitting fibers • Endomysium fibrosis • Rimmed vacuoles • NADH-TR: moth-eaten fibers • Reduced dystrophin stain • Reduced sarcoglycans • Reduced α-dystroglycans

Disease	Inheritance	Genetics	Clinical features	Investigations	Pathology
Facioscapulohumeral muscular dystrophy (FHMD)	ADD	**Type I**: DUX4 gene mutation on subtelomeric region of Ch.4q35 causes hypomethylation at the locus **Type II**: SMCHD1 gene mutation on Ch.18p11 **Both types cause D4Z4 DNA repeat hypomethylation and high expression of DUX4	• Usually adult onset • Progressive weakness of facial, shoulder, and limb-girdle muscles • Scapular winging • Dysarthria • Pectus excavatum • Associated with vascular retinopathy, hearing loss, or epilepsy • Cardiomyopathy	CK is ↑ EMG: myopathy NCT: non-specific Gene seq.	• Wide variation in fiber size • Dystrophy change • Minimal neuropathic change • Type II hypertrophy • Angulated fibers • Endomysium fibrosis • Minimal inflammation • MHC class I expression
Limb-girdle muscular dystrophy (LGMD)	**Type I** ADD **Type II** ARD	LGMD gene mutation on foci of chromosome encoded a specific related protein: **Type I** • 1A: TTID gene mutation on Ch.5q13 encoded myotilin (MFM) • 1B: LMNA gene mutation on Ch.1q21 encoded lamin A/C • 1C: Cave3 gene mutation on Ch.3p25 encoded caveolin-3 • 1D: DES gene mutation on Ch.2q35 encoded desmin (MFM-I) • 1E: DNAJB6 gene mutation on Ch.7q36 encoded DNAJB6 • 1F: TNPO3 gene on Ch.7q32 • 1G: HNRPDL gene mutation on Ch.4q21 **Type II** • 2A: CAPN3 mutation on Ch.15q15.1 encoded calpain-3 • 2B: DYSF gene mutation on Ch.2p13 encoded dysferlin (Miyoshi myopathy) • 2C: SG-G gene mutation on Ch.13q12 encoded sarcoglycan-γ • 2D: SG-A gene mutation on Ch.17q21 encoded sarcoglycan-α • 2E: SG-B gene mutation on Ch.4q12 encoded Sarcoglycan-β • 2F: SG-D on Ch.5q33 encoded sarcoglycan-δ; • 2G: TCAP gene mutation on Ch.17q12 encoded telethonin • 2H: Trim32 gene mutation on Ch.9q33 encoded tripartite • 2I: FKTN gene mutation on Ch.9q31 encoded FKRP • 2J: TTN gene on Ch.2q24 encoded titin • 2L: ANO5 gene on Ch.11p13 encoded anoctamin • 2X: POPDC3 gene mutation on Ch.6q21 encoded Popeye protein	• Late child or adult onset • Progressive muscle weakness of pelvis, limbs, and/or shoulder • Face is usually spared • Distal muscle wasting • Calf hypertrophy • Ankle contracture • Tip-toe walking (2B) • Scapular winging (2A/2F) • Lordosis • Dysarthria (1A) • Distal neuropathy (1A) • Dysphagia (1/7D) • AV block (1B) • SNHL in (2C) • Can be associated with cardiomyopathy • Mental retardation in early cases ** LGMD-2B can be misdiagnosed as polymyositis in early stage	CK is ↑ EMG: myopathy NCT: denervation **Others to do:** Potassium ↑ (2×) ECG Western blot Gene seq.	• Wide variation in fiber size • Myopathic changes • Type II hypertrophy • Multiple internal nuclei • Excessive splitting fibers • Few necrotic fibers • Basophilic or rounded fibers • Lobulated trabecular fibers • Endomysial fibrosis • Rimmed vacuoles 1A/1F/1E • COX (−) fibers in (1H) • Inflammation in (2B) (2J) • Amyloid deposition in (2B) • Neurogenic atrophy in (1A/1F) • MHC expression (2B) • Absent stains-related variants • Reduced α-dystroglycans (2I) EM: Myofibrillar disruption-Z line stream Autophagic vacuoles in (1/F). Nemaline rods in (1A).

(Continued)

Table 16.1. Muscular dystrophy diseases.

Disease	Pattern	Cause	Clinical features	Investigation	Microscopic Features
Emery-Dreifuss dystrophy (EDD)	Type I ARD Type II ADD Type III ARD Type IV ADD Type V XLD	Type I: STA gene mutation on Ch.Xq28 leads to absent emerin protein Type II/III: LMNA gene mutation on Ch.1q22 leads to absent lamin A/C protein (allelic with LGMD IB) Type IV: SYNE1 gene mutation on Ch.6q25 leads to reduced nesprin-1 protein Type V: FHL1 gene mutation on Ch.Xq26 leads to reduced FHL1 protein	• Child or adult onset • Neonatal hypotonia • Muscle weakness and wasting involve scapula, pelvis, and limbs • Scapular winging • Joints contracture • Camptocormia • Spine rigidity • Cardiac dysrhythmia • Cardiomyopathy • Lipodystrophy	CK is normal or ↑ EMG: myopathic NCT: non-specific	• Mild variation in fiber size • Myopathic/dystrophy change • Selective type I atrophy • Hypertrophic and round fibers • Multiple internal nuclei • Endomysial fibrosis • Fatty metaplasia • Rimmed vacuoles • Minimal inflammation • Neuromyopathic in type II/III • Absent emerin from all nuclei • Absent laminin β2 EM: Chromatin and nuclear detachment TFI

Congenital muscular dystrophy (CMD)

ARD

Group 1: Defect in sarcolemmal proteins – two variants:

A-Merosin deficiency syndrome: LAMA-2 gene mutation on Ch.6q lead to deficiency of laminin α2

B-Ulrich syndrome:
COL6A (1-2) genes mutation on Ch.21q22 lead to deficiency of collagen VI

Group 2: Dystroglycanopathies

A-Fukuyama CMD (FCMD):
FKTN gene mutation on Ch.9q31 lead to deficiency of fukutin protein (FKRP)—allelic with LGMD-2I

B-Muscle eye brain disease
POMGnT1 gene mutation on Ch.1p34 encodes
O-mannose-acetylglucosaminyltransferase

C-Walker–Warburg syndrome:
POMT1/2 gene mutation on Ch.9q34 or Ch.14q24 encodes
O-manosyltransferase

D-Rigid spine syndrome: SEPN1 gene mutation on Ch.1q36 leads to deficiency of selenoprotein N1

Group 3: CMD associated with mitochondrial abnormalities: CHKB gene mutation on Ch.22q13 leads to absent choline-kinase protein

- Usually birth onset
- Jewish or Japanese
- Generalized hypotonia
- Generalized weakness
- Developmental delay
- Spine rigidity
- Kyphoscoliosis
- Joint contractures

Association with group 1:
- Hyperlaxative joints
- Hyperkeratosis
- Epilepsy
- Hip dislocation
- White matter changes
- Mild neuropathy
- Cerebellar atrophy

Association with group 2:
- Mental retardation
- Nasal speech
- Scoliosis
- Epilepsy
- Hydrocephalus
- Ocular involvement
- Polymicrogyria
- Lissencephaly type II
- Occipital encephalocele
- Cerebellar hypoplasia
- Calf hypertrophy
- Scapular winging
- Cardiomyopathy

Association with group 3:
- Developmental delay
- Epilepsy
- Skin blistering
- Cardiomyopathy

- CK is ↑↑
- EMG: myopathic
- NCT: non-specific
Others to do:
- Brain MRI
- EEG
- Gene seq.

- Wide variation in fiber size
- Myopathic/dystrophic change
- Hypertrophic and round fibers
- Multiple internal nuclei
- Excessive splitting fibers
- Endomysial fibrosis
- Minimal inflammation (1A)
- Lobulated fibers (1B)
- Reduced laminin α2 (1A)
- Reduced merosin (1A)
- Reduced collagen VI (1B)
- Reduced dystrophin (2A)
- Increased laminin β2 (2B)
- Minicores (2D)
- Reduced α-dystroglycans in all group 2 diseases
- Reduced COX in group 3

EM:
- Myofibrillar disruption
- Abnormal mitochondria in G3
- Disorganized collagen (1B)
- Sarcomere defect (2D)

(Continued)

Table 16.1. Muscular dystrophy diseases. (Continued)

Disease	Pattern		Cause	Clinical features	Investigation	Microscopic Features
Bethlem myopathy	ADD ARD		COL6A (1-3) genes mutation (exon 3-14) on Ch.21q22 or Ch.2q37 encodes collagen VI protein. Allelic with Ulrich syndrome	• Usually early child onset • Neonatal hypotonia • Joint contracture • Proximal > distal weakness • Waddling gait • Finger flexor contracture • Hypertrophic scar • Failed prayer sign	CK is ↑ EMG: myopathy NCT: non-specific **Others to do:** US: central cloud	• Dystrophic change • Myopathic change • Multiple ring fibers • Core-like fibers • Reduced laminin β1 • Normal collagen VI labeling
Scapuloperoneal muscular dystrophy (hyaline body myopathy) (myosin storage myopathy)	**Type I** ADD **Type II** ARD **Type III** ADD		**Type I:** FHL-1 gene mutation on Ch.Xq26 leads to reduced four and a half LIM protein **Type II/III:** MYH-7 gene mutation on Ch.14q11 leads to storage of myosin heavy chain ****Other variants:** Scapuloperoneal neuropathy due to TRPV4 or TRIM32 gene mutations	• Adult onset • Italian families • Proximal muscle weakness and wasting • Scapuloperoneal muscle weakness (bent spine) • Scapular winging • Peripheral neuropathy • Hearing loss • Cardiomyopathy	CK is ↑ EMG: myopathic NCT: non-specific	• Mild variation in fiber size • Focal myopathic change • Fatty infiltration • Hypertrophic fibers • Endomysial fibrosis • Hyaline body; subsarcolemmal hyaline areas in type I>II fibers (+ for desmin, FHL-1 and dystrophin stains) • Desmin aggregation
Myotonic dystrophy	ADD		Trinucleotide repeat expansion (CTG) > 20 times on terminal end of exon 15. **Two types:** **Type I** (Steinert disease): DMPK gene mutation on Ch.19q13 leads to reduced myotonin kinase protein causing Na channel defect and expanded CUG RNA repeat **Type II** (Proximal dystrophy): ZNF9 gene mutation on Ch.3q21 lead to low zinc finger protein 9, less severe clinical form than type I	• Young-adult onset • Can be congenital • Proximal > distal muscle weakness and wasting with myotonia I > II • Bilateral ptosis • Frontal baldness • Temporalis wasting • Hypersomnia • Dysphagia • Can be associated with diabetes, dysrhythmia, cataract, gonadal atrophy	CK is ↑ Serum IgG low EMG: myopathic, waxing and waning repetitive stimuli **Others to do:** Brain MRI Genetic test	• Wide variation in fiber size • Type I fiber atrophy in I > II • Type II hypertrophy in II > I • Type I fiber predominance • Endomysium fibrosis • Numerous internal nuclei • Pyknotic nuclear clump • Multiple splitting fibers • Ring and targetoid fibers **EM:** Irregular myonuclei Myofibrillar disruption Dilated sarcoplasmic reticulum

| Oculopharyngeal muscular dystrophy (OPMD) | ADD ARD | Trinucleotide repeat expansion (GCG or GCA) > 13 times on exon 1, due to PABPN-1/2 gene mutation on Ch.14q.11 **Note:**
• PABPN-1 functions as polyadenylation of mRNA.
• Oculopharyngeal distal myopathy should be excluded | • Adult onset
• French Canadian
• Bilateral ptosis
• Opthalmoplagia
• Dysphagia
• Generalized weakness
• Astrologist neck
• Neuropathy | CK is ↑
EMG: myopathic or denervation | • Wide variation in fiber size
• Dystrophy change
• Type II hypertrophy
• Angulated fibers (+NADH)
• Rimmed vacuoles
• Cytoplasmic bodies
• Few cores devoid COX/SDH
• Rare ragged red fibers
• Ubiquitin positive inclusions
__EM:__ Rimmed vacuoles-TFI-Nuclear clearing-cytoplasmic body-Finger print bodies |

Abbreviations: XLR: X-lined recessive. ADD: autosomal dominant disease. ARD: autosomal recessive disease. CK: creatinine kinase. EMG: electromyography. ECD: echocardiogram. AST: aspartate aminotransferase. ALT: alanine transaminase. SNHL: sensorineural hearing loss. EEG: electroencephalogram. EM: electron microscopy. DUX4: double homeobox 4. TTID: titin immunoglobin domain. LMNA: lamin A/C. DNABJ6: DNA heat shock protein family member B6. TRIM32: tripartite motif containing 32. FKRP: fukutin-related protein. ANOS: anoctamin 5. SYNE1: spectrin repeat containing nuclear envelope protein 1. FHL1: four and a half LIM domains protein 1. POMGnT1: protein O-linked mannose N-acetylglucosaminyltransferase 1. SEPN1: selenoprotein 1. TRPV4: transient receptor potential cation channel subfamily V member 4. DMPK: DM1 protein kinase. CTG: cytosine-thymine-guanine. ZNF9: zink finger protein 9. MRI: magnetic resonance imaging. PABPN1: polyadenylate binding protein nuclear 1 gene (polyalanine). TFI: tubulofilamentous inclusions. mRNA: messenger RNA.

of a family, while facioscapulohumeral dystrophy (FHMD) has an autosomal dominant pattern. The gold standard diagnostic method to differentiate between dystrophies is genetic testing. Almost 30 genes and encoded proteins are known to be associated with different dystrophy diseases.

Duchenne muscular dystrophy (DMD) was recognized as a clinical entity in the nineteenth century. It is considered one of the common muscular disorders in clinical practice. With **Becker muscular dystrophy** (BMD) and DMD both share the same gene mutation and encoded protein defect. **Table 16.1** explains the definition, gene mutations, clinical features, investigational findings, and muscle histology of these two entities.

The classical histological feature of any myopathic dystrophy is almost similar. The main solid feature is the presence of myopathic change with marked fibrosis. Diffuse variation in fiber size and shape with alternative muscle fiber atrophy, hypertrophy, and rounding fibers are always seen. There is also minimal necrosis and regeneration. The endomysial connective tissue is always thickened and fibrotic (**Figure 16.1**). Splitting fibers and moth-eaten fibers are common histological features in dystrophy diseases. Some dystrophic diseases may show additional remarkable changes such as focal inflammation in LGMD-2B and rimmed vacuoles in some LGMDs, BMD, or oculopharyngeal muscular dystrophy (OPMD). Because of sarcolemmal protein interaction between muscle diseases, careful interpretation of muscle protein deficiencies should be taken into account.

It is impossible to distinguish DMD or BMD from other muscular dystrophies on the basis of histology alone. Histochemical reaction and genetic testing are mandating. The dystrophin gene is considered one of the largest gene defects in the MD group. Its protein is located in the sarcoplasmic

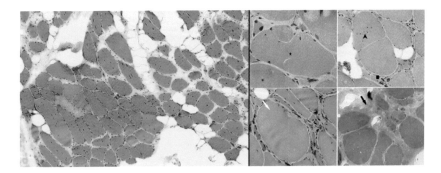

Figure 16.1 Histological features of Myopathic Dystrophy. The four small images in the right-side show splitting fiber (*); multiple internal nuclei (*arrow head*); pyknotic nuclear clumps (*black square*); hypertrophic fiber surrounded by small atrophic fibers (*white arrow*); endomysial fibrosis on GT stain (*black arrow*).

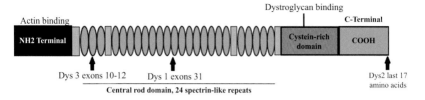

Figure 16.2 Dystrophin gene with its four domains (cysteine, C-terminal, NH2-terminal, and central rod domain).

membrane interacting with sarcoglycans and dystroglycans (see *Figure 1.3 in Chapter 1, Part I*). The gene has four domains with exons, illustrated in **Figure 16.2**. About two-thirds of identified mutations in the *dystrophin* gene are deletions, about one-third are point mutations, and a small proportion are duplications (**Table 16.1**). Point mutations are difficult to identify with a polymerase chain reaction (PCR) but immunohistochemistry (IHC) can easily identify all mutations that led to a stop codon and result in protein absence.

It is unreliable to make a diagnosis of DMD or BMD based only on molecular analysis, emphasizing the need to examine protein expression in muscle tissue. Complete absence of dystrophin stain in all muscle fibers remains diagnostic for DMD (**Figure 16.3**). If the protein is reduced in some muscle fibers and the patient is a woman, or a man with milder symptoms, the defective gene could be a carrier. Manifesting carriers invariably show some fibers that lack dystrophin expression. In asymptomatic carriers, few changes in dystrophin expression are detectable or literally negative. If the histological abnormalities from a female muscle are remarkable but dystrophin immunolabelling appears normal, the patient is unlikely to be a carrier. Bear in mind that some regenerating and immature fibers can also show low dystrophin expression. Therefore, careful interpretation of stain results are important to avoid any diagnostic error. Spectrin, sarcoglycans, and dystroglycans can all be used as positive controls.

Because of the mutational variability in the *dystrophin* gene, it is essential to use antibodies that correspond to more than one domain; to avoid any false-negative result. Very low levels of dystrophin expression can be detected in some DMD cases, probably from minor transcripts of the gene. It is recently thought to result from exon skipping.

Finally, DMD and BMD are considered one disease with variable features. The diagnosis requires careful reading of muscle histology and protein expression.

Limb-girdle muscular dystrophies (LGMDs) are a group of inherited disorders with either autosomal dominant or autosomal recessive patterns.

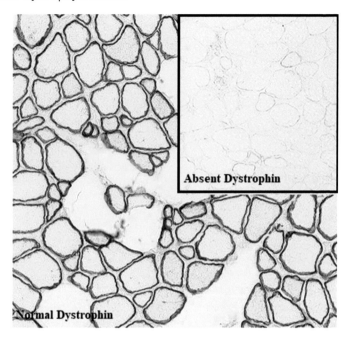

Figure 16.3 Histological sections from a 16-year-old boy with Duchenne muscular dystrophy (DMD) show absent dyst-2 protein immunolabelling in the sarcolemma, with normal positive control. ×25.

Dominant forms have been classified as LGMD-type I while recessive forms have been categorized as LGMD-type II. Each form has different gene mutations and particular protein defects (**Table 16.1**). The clinical features and investigational findings of all LGMD variants are similar. Although both groups affect the limb-girdle and shoulder muscles, they cannot be taken as diagnosing features for LGMD.

The classical histological features of LGMDs are similar to other types of dystrophies, such as DMD and BMD. However, it was commonly observed that excessive splitting fibers are predominant features in most LGMDs. It is actually not possible to distinguish LGMD from DMD or BMD based on muscle histology alone. Indeed, IHC and genetic analysis are essential. Immunolabeling-based diagnosis in LGMDs clarifies which gene and encoded protein is affected. Some of these diseases can overlap with other myopathic diseases. For example, LGMD-1A has the same overlapping protein defect seen in MFM. Moreover, LGMD-1D is genetically similar to MFM-type I (desminopathy). There is also a clear overlap between LGMD-1B and autosomal dominant Emery–Dreifuss dystrophy (EDD)-type II/III. All these clinical and morphological overlaps would not affect the patient diagnosis, prognosis, or management.

LGMD-2B (Miyoshi myopathy) is one of the most common variants among all LGMD groups. The predominant feature is the presence of focal inflammation. It is difficult sometimes to differentiate it from inflammatory myositis, especially if the morphological features are fuzzy. Although MHC class-I expression has been detected in few published cases of LGMD-2B, many pathologists still use MHC class-I to differentiate LGMD-2B from inflammatory myositis.

The second most common LGMD is sarcoglycanopathies (LGMD2C-F). LGMD-2C is the worst and most severe form, and its morphological and clinical phenotype are close to DMD. In pathology practice, a total absence or reduction of sarcoglycan in one or more than one muscle fibers is indicative of sarcoglycanopathy. The dystrophin protein is always normal in these cases.

Congenital muscular dystrophy (CMD) is described as a group of autosomal recessive muscular dystrophy affecting infants in their early life and associated with delayed milestone, hypotonia, and progressive muscle weakness and atrophy. These disorders are quite different from DMD, BMD, or LGMD as they have congenital origin and specific gene mutations. Further clinical studies combined with molecular inputs have revolutionized this field into a novel pathogenic mechanism in muscle that involves structural protein modification by glycosylation. It has recently been recognized as a separate pathological entity.

Because the muscle tissue appearance of these cases is child muscle, the histological features are sometimes subtle and cannot lead to a specific diagnosis. Older children may show features of myopathic dystrophy that were mentioned earlier. CMD is classified into four groups, described in **Table 16.1**. Although Bethlem myopathy is considered a congenital dystrophy type, it has also been reported in older children and young people. Bear in mind that CMD is always a birth-onset and progresses over life to worse conditions. Pathologists can never diagnose CMD by only clinical history and histology. The muscle histology may show unremarkable or minimal non-specific change. IHC is essential for the analysis of all cases of CMD to visualize and localize the deficient proteins.

The most common types of CMD are group 1 (**Table 16.1**). Because their antibodies are commercially available, the diagnosis can be made through IHC. In collage VI deficiency (Ulrich syndrome), the collagen immunolabeling pattern is always weak. Because Ulrich syndrome and Bethlem myopathy are closely related in clinical ground, the effect of a particular mutation on the production and function of collagen VI may determine the severity. In general, the immunolabeling pattern of collagen VI is always unequivocal or may show some reduction. Nevertheless, collagen VI could be normal in Bethlem myopathy. To help differentiate Ulrich from Bethlem myopathies, Lamin B1 is used commonly as a secondary labeling index in Bethlem myopathy, which shows a reduction in staining pattern.

Dystroglycanopathies are a rare group of CMD. They are associated with hypoglycosylation of dystroglycans. A secondary reduction of α- or β-dystroglycan has also been observed in cases with DMD and BMD.

CMD group 1, Bethlem myopathy and Emery-Dreifuss dystrophy (EDD) all share slightly similar clinical and morphological features in muscle biopsy. However, EDD is commonly associated with joint contracture. Several variants with different inheritance patterns are categorized under EDD (**Table 16.1**). Because the pathological features of EDD resemble all types of muscular dystrophies, IHC is considered the best differential tool to detect the protein deficiency. Emerin and lamin are commercially available antibodies and their sensitivity and specificity are high (**Figure 16.4**).

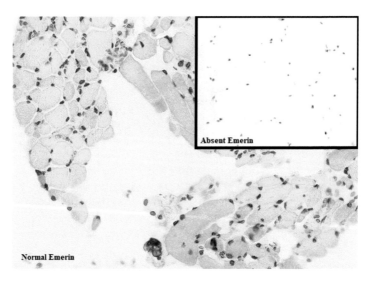

Figure 16.4 Histological sections from a 21-year-old man with Emery-Dreifuss dystrophy (EDD) show absent emerin immunolabeling in the muscle nuclei, with normal positive control. ×25.

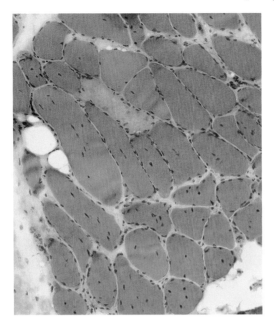

Figure 16.5 H&E section from a patient with myotonic dystrophy. There is myonecrosis with multiple internal nuclei in every single muscle fiber. ×25.

In conclusion, we can say that all cases suspected for CMD should undergo genetic analysis.

Facioscapulohumeral muscular dystrophy (FHMD), **myotonic dystrophy** (DM), and **oculopharyngeal muscular dystrophy** (OPMD) are autosomal dominant disorders of unusual molecular defect that involve nucleotide repeats. The characteristic features are similar, and their diagnoses cannot be made on muscle biopsy alone. No specific pathological features or IHC findings have been identified in affected patients of FHMD despite previous published studies.

In DM, myotonia in both type I and type II variants differs in the pattern of muscle weakness. In type II, there is early proximal muscle involvement, in contrast to the distal pattern seen in type I. Some literature has differentiated type I from type II variants through histological features. This is inaccurate and has no basis. However, the most predominant feature to say this case is DM is the presence of multiple internal nuclei in every single muscle fiber (**Figure 16.5**). Otherwise, IHC studies or electron microscopy (EM) would

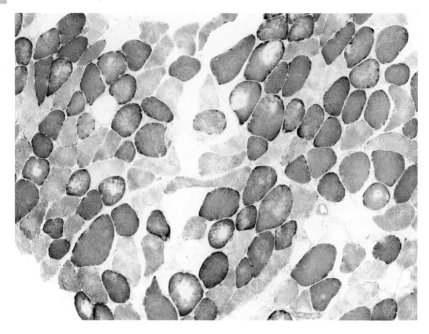

Figure 16.6 COX stain on a muscle section of a patient with OPMD showing fibers with core-like lesions; a common finding in OPMD cases.

not help in the diagnosis. The muscle pathology in congenital myotonic dystrophy is characteristic as many fibers have large central nuclei with a pale peripheral halo; this resembles centronuclear myopathy. In this case, diagnosis is difficult to establish. Molecular analysis is the best tool to differentiate between these entities.

OPMD is characterized histologically by dystrophic features, rare ragged red fibers, rare rimmed vacuoles, cytoplasmic bodies, and many fibers with core-like lesions. Core-like lesions of muscle fibers in COX stain are a common finding in these cases (**Figure 16.6**).

In summary, muscular dystrophy is characterized clinically and histologically with myopathic features, dystrophic pattern, and muscle fibrosis. Pathologists should do the usual and common panel of dystrophy proteins. The panel rarely shows protein deficiency; however, molecular analysis is important for the final diagnosis.

CLINICAL CASE

A 23-year-old man presented to the neuromuscular clinic with only progressive weakness of limb-girdle muscles. The patient occasionally walks on his tip-toes. There is no typical history of such presentation in his family. Neurological examination demonstrates weak biceps and quadriceps muscles with normal reflexes. Mild calf hypertrophy is noted as well. There is no remarkable sensory disturbance.

Serum CK level is elevated (6000 IU/L). EMG demonstrates spontaneous activity, early recruitment, and small motor unit potential. Normal sensory nerve conduction study is also observed on NCT.

Based on the Above Findings, What is Your Differential Diagnosis?

A biopsy is done from the right deltoid muscle. Sections treated with H&E, dystrophy immunolabeling panel including dysferlin (**Figure 16.7**).

- Explain the histopathological findings.
- What is your likely diagnosis?

Interpretation

H&E section shows minimal myopathic features, multiple splitting fibers, few internal nuclei, and endomysial fibrosis. There is a focal inflammation (**Figure 16.7a**). MHC class-I is expressed only in the vasculature. Sarcolemmal dystrophy immunolabeling is normally present in the muscle fibers except dysferlin stain, which shows total negative staining (**Figure 16.7b**). These features are consistent with the diagnosis of Limb-girdle muscular dystrophy (LGMD-type 2B). Genetic testing is recommended to confirm the diagnosis.

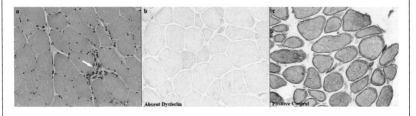

Figure 16.7 Histological sections from a 23-year-old man presenting with limb-girdle muscle weakness. **(a)** H&E section shows minimal myopathic dystrophy change and a focal inflammation (*white arrow*). **(b)** Absent dysferlin immunolabeling. **(c)** Normal positive control of dysferlin stain. ×25.

References

Anderson LV, Harrison RM, Pogue R, et al. Secondary reduction in calpain 3 expression in patients with limb girdle muscular dystrophy type 2B and Miyoshi myopathy (primary dysferlinopathies). Neuromuscul Disord. 2000; 10: 553–559.

Arikawa E, Ishihara T, Nonaka I, et al. Immunocytochemical analysis of dystrophin in congenital muscular dystrophy. J Neurol Sci. 1991; 105: 79–87.

Askanas V, Serdaroglu P, Engel WK, et al. Immunolocalization of ubiquitin in muscle biopsies of patients with inclusion body myositis and oculopharyngeal muscular dystrophy. Neurosci Lett. 1991; 130: 73–76.

Ben Yaou R, Toutain A, Arimura T, et al. Multitissular involvement in a family with LMNA and EMD mutations: role of digenic mechanism? Neurology. 2007; 68: 1883–1894.

Bengoechea R, Tapia O, Casafont I, et al. Nuclear speckles are involved in nuclear aggregation of PABPN1 and in the pathophysiology of oculopharyngeal muscular dystrophy. Neurobiol Dis. 2012; 46: 118–129.

Bertini E, D'Amico A, Gualandi F, et al. Congenital muscular dystrophies: a brief review. Semin Pediatr Neurol. 2011; 18: 277–288.

Brais B, Rouleau GA, Bouchard JP, Fardeau M, Tome FM. Oculopharyngeal muscular dystrophy. Semin Neurol. 1999; 19: 59–66.

Brockington M, Blake DJ, Prandini P, et al. Mutations in the fukutin-related protein gene (FKRP) cause a form of congenital muscular dystrophy with secondary laminin alpha2 deficiency and abnormal glycosylation of alphadystroglycan. Am J Hum Genet. 2001; 69: 1198–1209.

Broglio L, Tentorio M, Cotelli MS, et al. Limb-girdle muscular dystrophy-associated protein diseases. Neurologist. 2010; 16: 340–352.

Brown SC, Lucy JA. Dystrophin: gene, protein and cell biology. Cambridge University Press, Cambridge. 1997.

Carango P, Noble JE, Marks HG, Funanage VL. Absence of myotonic dystrophy protein kinase (DMPK) mRNA as a result of a triplet repeat expansion in myotonic dystrophy. Genomics. 1993; 18: 340–348.

Clerk A, Rodillo E, Heckmatt JZ, et al. Characterisation of dystrophin in carriers of Duchenne muscular dystrophy. J Neurol Sci. 1991; 102: 197–205.

Di Blasi C, Morandi L, Raffaele di Barletta M, et al. Unusual expression of emerin in a patient with X-linked Emery-Dreifuss muscular dystrophy. Neuromuscul Disord. 2000; 10: 567–571.

Dickey RP, Ziter FA, Smith RA. Emery-Dreifuss muscular dystrophy. J Pediat. 1984; 104: 555–559.

Dincer P, Balci B, Yuva Y, et al. A novel form of recessive limb girdle muscular dystrophy with mental retardation and abnormal expression of alpha-dystroglycan. Neuromuscul Disord. 2003; 13: 771–778.

Dubowitz V. Rigid spine syndrome: a muscle syndrome in search of a name. Proc R Soc Med. 1973; 66: 219–220.

Ferreiro A, Mezmezian M, Olive M, et al. Telethonin deficiency initially presenting as a congenital muscular dystrophy. Neuromuscul Disord. 2011; 21: 433–438.

Fitzsimons RB. Retinal vascular disease and the pathogenesis of facioscapulohumeral muscular dystrophy. A signaling message from Wnt? Neuromuscul Disord. 2011; 21: 263–271.

Flanigan KM, Von Niederhausern A, Dunn DM, et al. Rapid direct sequence analysis of the dystrophin gene. Am J Hum Genet. 2003; 72(4): 931–939.

Fulizio L, Nascimbeni AC, Fanin M, Piluso G, et al. Molecular and muscle pathology in a series of caveolinopathy patients. Hum Mutat. 2005; 25: 82–89.

Gayathri N, Alefia R, Nalini A, et al. Dysferlinopathy: spectrum of pathological changes in skeletal muscle tissue. Indian J Pathol Microbiol. 2011; 54: 350–354.

Godfrey C, Foley AR, Clement E, et al. Dystroglycanopathies: coming into focus. Curr Opin Genet Dev. 2011; 21: 278–285.

Gualandi F, Urciuolo A, Martoni E, et al. Autosomal recessive Bethlem myopathy. Neurology. 2009; 73: 1883–1891.

Harms MB, Sommerville RB, Allred P, et al. Exome sequencing reveals DNAJB6 mutations in dominantly inherited myopathy. Ann Neurol. 2012; 71: 407–416.

Helliwell TR, Nguyen TM, Morris GE. The dystrophin-related protein, utrophin, is expressed on the sarcolemma of regenerating human skeletal muscle fibers in dystrophies and inflammatory myopathies. Neuromuscul Disord. 1992; 2: 177–184.

Hewitt JE, Lyle R, Clark LN, Valleley EM, et al. Analysis of the tandem repeat locus D4Z4 associated with facioscapulohumeral muscular dystrophy. Hum Molec Genet. 1994; 3: 1287–1295.

Kamei D, Tsuchiya N, Yamazaki M, Meguro H, Yamada M. Two forms of expression and genomic structure of the human heterogeneous nuclear ribonucleoprotein D-like JKTBP gene (HNRPDL). Gene. 1999; 228: 13–22.

Kirschner J, Hausser I, Zou Y, et al. Ullrich congenital muscular dystrophy: connective tissue abnormalities in the skin support overlap with Ehlers–Danlos syndromes. Am J Med Genet A. 2005; 132: 296–301.

Kondo E, Saito K, Osawa M. Muscular dystrophy. Nihon Rinsho. 2005; 63(3): 420–428.

Lemmers RJ, Tawil R, Petek LM, Balog J, Block GJ, at al. Digenic inheritance of an SMCHD1 mutation and an FSHD-permissive D4Z4 allele causes facioscapulohumeral muscular dystrophy type 2. Nat Genet. 2012; 44(12): 1370–1374.

Machuca-Tzili L, Brook D, Hilton-Jones D. Clinical and molecular aspects of the myotonic dystrophies: a review. Muscle Nerve. 2005; 32: 1–18.

Melia MJ, Kubota A, Ortolano S, Vilchez JJ, Gamez J, Tanji K, et al. Limb-girdle muscular dystrophy 1F is caused by a microdeletion in the transportin 3 gene. Brain. 2013; 136: 1508–1517.

Michele DE, Campbell KP. Dystrophin-glycoprotein complex: post-translational processing and dystroglycan function. J Biol Chem. 2003; 278: 15457–15460.

Morris GE. The role of the nuclear envelope in Emery-Dreifuss muscular dystrophy. Trends Mol Med. 2001; 7(12): 572–527.

Muntoni F, Torelli S, Wells DJ, et al. Muscular dystrophies due to glycosylation defects: diagnosis and therapeutic strategies. Curr Opin Neurol. 2011; 24: 437–442.

Naom I, D'Alessandro M, Sewry C, et al. The role of immunocytochemistry and linkage analysis in the prenatal diagnosis of merosin-deficient congenital muscular dystrophy. Hum Genet. 1997; 99: 535–540.

Orrel RW. Diagnosing and managing muscular dystrophy. Practitioner. 2012; 256(1754): 21–24,2–3.

Quinzii CM, Vu TH, Min KC, Tanji K, Barral S, et al. X-linked dominant scapuloperoneal myopathy is due to mutation in the gene encoding four-and-a-half-LIM protein 1. Am J Hum Genet. 2008; 82: 208–213.

Rosales XQ, Gastier-Foster JM, Lewis S, et al. Novel diagnostic features of dysferlinopathy. Muscle Nerve. 2010; 42: 14–21.

Satoyoshi E, Kinoshita M. Oculopharyngodistal myopathy. Arch Neurol. 1977; 34: 89–92.

Sewry CA, Brown SC, Mercuri E, et al. Skeletal muscle pathology in autosomal dominant Emery–Dreifuss muscular dystrophy with lamin A/C mutations. Neuropathol Appl Neurobiol. 2001; 27: 281–290.

Statland JM, Tawil R. Facioscapulohumeral muscular dystrophy: molecular pathological advances and future directions. Curr Opin Neurol. 2011; 24: 423–428.

Vihola A, Bassez G, Meola G, et al. Histopathological differences of myotonic dystrophy type 1 (DM1) and PROMM/DM2. Neurology. 2003; 60: 1854–1857.

Yin Xi, Wang Qian, Chen T, at al. CD4 cells, macrophages, MHC-I, and C5v-o involve the pathogenesis of dysferlinopathy. Int J Clin Exp Pathol. 2015; 8(3): 3069–3075.

CHAPTER 17
INHERITED MYOPATHIC DISEASES

Inherited myopathic diseases are a diverse group of neuromuscular disorders characterized by unique histopathological features and specific genetic abnormalities. Some of these diseases have been mentioned in previous chapters as part of other diagnostic approaches such as the conditions described in vacuolar myopathy or neuromyopathies. (See *Chapters 14* and *15*). Diagnosis of these disorders is contingent on clinical history and physical examination, muscle biopsy, and genetic testing.

The clinical presentation does not often occur at birth; some cases reported late-adulthood presentation. This could make the diagnosis more difficult in clinical ground. The most common clinical feature at birth is generalized hypotonia and isolated developmental delay. A slowly progressive muscle weakness or cramps are common in adulthood. Some cases present with weakness at limb-girdle muscle distribution. Of the inherited myopathies, 10% to 20% are associated with structural abnormalities in several systemic organs. Asymptomatic patients or carriers account for 5% to 10%.

Serum CK level and electrophysiological studies may not literally help in the differential diagnosis. In these cases, muscle biopsy is indicated. Advances in molecular studies have led to the identification of many genetic mutations associated with these congenital myopathies.

Inherited myopathic diseases include any abnormal neuromuscular condition not belonging to muscular dystrophy groups, acquired myopathies, or inflammatory myopathies. Some of these conditions can be diagnosed through muscle biopsy. Some pathological features are unique for particular disorders and all are consequences of specific gene mutations. However, the need for molecular analysis is important to identify these mutant genes.

Table 17.1 summarizes the inherited myopathic diseases most commonly seen in clinicopathological practice.

Core myopathy or **central core disease** (CCD) is one of the most common congenital myopathies in neurological practice. Patients clinically present with non-progressive muscle weakness. Rare cases were found to be associated with malignant hyperthermia and some other variants summarized in **Table 17.1**. The disease is histologically characterized by the presence of structural or non-structural

Table 17.1 Inherited myopathic diseases not part of muscular dystrophy or other acquired myopathies.

Disease	Pattern	Cause	Clinical features	Investigation	Microscopic features
Central core myopathy (CCD)	ADD ARD	RYR-1 gene mutation on Ch.19q13 "C-terminal exons 95-102" encodes Ryanodine receptor protein of calcium channel, damaging the gap between SR and T-tubule. 80% missense mutation. Variants: • Malignant hyperthermia • King-Denborough syndrome • Limb-girdle syndrome • Nemaline rod myopathy • Exertional rhabdomyolysis • Centronuclear myopathy • Adult-onset axial myopathy (Bent spine syndrome)	• Usually childhood onset • Can be adult onset • Developmental delay • Generalized hypotonia • Non-progressive lower limb muscle weakness • Generalized cramps • Mild facial weakness • Associated with hip dislocation or scoliosis • Can be associated with malignant hyperthermia, scoliosis, and bent spine (camptocormia)	CK is normal EMG: myopathic NCT: non-specific Others to do: Spine MRI Genetic Seq.	• Mild variation in fiber size • Myopathic change • Type I fiber predominance • Endomysial fibrosis • Multiple central cores, more in type I than type II fibers • Cores express desmin and β-crystalline but devoid RYR1 and oxidative stains • Multiple central nuclei EM: • Myofibrillar disruption • Cores (structured/non) devoid mitochondria and SR • Cores containing rods • Z-line streaming
Minicore myopathy (MCM)	ARD	Type I: RYR-1 gene mutation on Ch.19q13 encodes ryanodine receptor protein Type II: SEPN1 gene mutation on Ch.1p36.11 encodes selenoprotein N1	• Child or adult onset • Developmental delay • Generalized hypotonia • Non-progressive muscle weakness; axial>limbs • Spinal rigidity • Mild facial weakness • Can be associated with ophthalmoplegia, scoliosis, cardiac disease	CK is normal EMG: myopathic NCT: non-specific	• Mild variation in fiber size • Myopathic change • Multiple internal nuclei • Type I fiber predominance • Multiple minicores • Cores express desmin and β-crystalline but devoid oxidative stains EM: Myofibrillar disruption and cores devoid mitochondria
Nemaline rod myopathy (NRM)	ADD ARD	Type I: ACTA1 gene mutation on Ch.1q42 encodes α-Actin Type II: NEB gene mutation on Ch.2q2 encodes nebulin Type III: TPM2 gene mutation on Ch9q13 encodes tropomyosin-B Type IV: TNNT1 gene mutation on Ch.19q13 encodes troponin T1	• Child onset (type II) • Late adult (SLONM) • Generalized weakness • Floppy baby syndrome • Dysmorphism • High-arched palate • Rigid spine or scoliosis • Respiratory dysfunction • Can be associated with cardiomyopathy and MGUS	CK is normal or ↑ EMG: myopathic NCT: non-specific Genetic Seq.	• Wide variation in fiber size • Myopathic change • Small type I fibers • Type I predominance • Glycogen accumulation • Fibers with core-like lesions • GT stain: multiple nemaline rods (green-blue) EM: • Myofibrillar disruption • Electron dense rods parallel to sarcomere • Whorling actin-band and thick Z-line

Disease	Inheritance	Genetics	Clinical	Investigations	Histology / EM
Myotubular myopathy (centronuclear myopathy)	**Type I** XLR **Type II** ADD **Type III** ARD	**Type I:** MTM1 gene mutation on Ch. Xq28 encodes myotubularin protein, found in the I-band and express ubiquitin. • 50% point mutation • 30% insertion or deletion • Germline mosaicism in female **Type II:** CNM1 (DNM2) gene mutation on Ch. 19p13 encodes Dynamin 2 protein **Type III:** CNM2 gene mutation on Ch.2q14 encodes bridging integrator-1 protein	• Child onset • Adult onset (type II) • Male > female • Developmental delay • Generalized hypotonia • Generalized weakness • Mild facial weakness • High-arched palate • Opthalmoparesis • Respiratory failure • Cardiomyopathy • Can be associated with scoliosis, renal stones, and hepatic dysfunction	CK is normal or ↑ EMG: myopathic NCT: non-specific RNA seq.	• Mild variation in fiber size • Minimal myopathic change • Scattered necrotic fibers • Endomysial fibrosis • Type I fiber predominance • Central pallor on ATPase • Large central internal nuclei • Perinuclear vacuoles devoid NADH, COX, and GT staining • Multiple ring fibers **EM:** Myofibrillar disruption, large internal nuclei, and central accumulation of mitochondria and glycogens
Myofibrillar myopathies (MFM)	ADD ARD	**Type I:** Desminopathy; due to DES gene mutation on ch.2q35 encodes Desmin protein, allelic with LGMD-1E **Type II:** αB-Crystalinopathy; due to CRYAB gene mutation on Ch.11q22 encodes β-crystalline **Type III:** Myotilinopathy; due to MYOT gene mutation on Ch.5q31 encodes myotilin protein, allelic with LGMD-1A **Type IV:** Zaspinopathy; due to ZASP gene mutation on Ch.10q22 encodes Z-band spliced PDZ-motif protein **Type V:** Filaminopathy; due to FLNC gene mutation on Ch.7q32 encodes filamin C protein **Type VI:** Bag3opathy; due to BAG3 gene mutation on Ch.10q25 encodes BCL-2 associated athanogene 3 (Bag3) **Type VII:** FHL1opathy; due to FHL1 mutation on Ch.Xq26.3 encodes FHL1 protein, XLD	• Child or adult onset • German races in type V • Non-progressive muscle weakness and wasting proximal > distal • **Type I/II** associated with cataract and peripheral neuropathy • **Type III/IV** associated with opthalmoplagia and peripheral neuropathy • **Type IV/V** associated with distal myopathy and peripheral neuropathy • Dysphagia in **type II** • Scapular winging • Can be associated with cardiomyopathy, cardiac block, or respiratory failure (HMERF disease)	CK is normal or ↑ EMG: myopathic with myotonia NCT: neuropathic **Others to do:** ECG Gene Seq.	• Mild variation in fiber size • Myopathic change • Neuromyopathic change • Necrosis and regeneration • Few internal nuclei • Wiped out areas (core-like) • Autophagic vacuoles • Rimmed vacuoles • Eosinophilic aggregates • Cytoplasmic bodies • Protein aggregates stain dark blue on GT • Aggregate of β-crystalline, ubiquitin, desmin, filamin, dystrophin, or myotullin stain • Myofibrillar apparatus • Amyloid deposition • Rare ragged red fibers • Rare Cox (–) negative fibers • Neuropathic changes mainly seen in **type IV/V** **EM:** • Myofibrillar disruption • Z-line streaming • Granulofilamentous materials • Cytoplasmic bodies

(Continued)

Table 17.1 Inherited myopathic diseases not part of muscular dystrophy or other acquired myopathies. (Continued)

Disease	Pattern	Cause	Clinical features	Investigation	Microscopic features
Tubular aggregate myopathy (TAM)	Sporadic ADD	**Type I:** STIM1 gene mutation on Ch.11p15 encodes stromal interaction molecule **Type II:** ORAI gene mutation on Ch.12q24 encodes orai calcium release calcium modulator ****TAM can be associated with myositis, hypokalemic periodic paralysis, myotonic syndrome, and malignant hyperthermia	• Young or adult onset • Slowly progressive proximal weakness • Muscle cramps • Quadriceps atrophy • Miosis in type II • Opthalmoplegia	CK is normal or ↑ EMG: myopathic NCT: non-specific **Others to do:** Low platelets Potassium level Gene Seq.	• Wide variation in fiber size • Myopathic change • Type II atrophy • Tubular aggregate with slits in type II>I: basophilic with cracks on H&E, red-green on GT, dark blue on NADH, clear on SDH/ATPase. • RYR1 aggregates EM hexagonal tubules arranged in honeycomb appearance 50–70 nm
Titinopathy	ADD ARD	TTN gene mutation on Ch.2q31. encodes titin protein. ****Can be allelic and associated with the following variants:** • Tibial dystrophy "LGMD-2J" • Centronuclear myopathy • Cytoplasmic body myopathy • Hereditary myopathy with respiratory failure (HMRF) • Fiber type disproportion • Emery-Dreifuss dystrophy variant	• Child or adult onset • Always Finnish/French • Generalized hypotonia • Distal muscle weakness • Cardiomyopathy • Scapular winging Calf pseudohypertrophy • Spinal rigidity • Respiratory failure	CK is ↑ EMG: myopathic NCT: non-specific	• Mild variation in fiber size • Myopathic change • Scattered necrotic fibers • Hypoplastic immature fibers • Multiple internal nuclei • Rimmed vacuoles • Protein aggregates • Cytoplasmic bodies • Absent Calpain-3 stain EM: abnormal M-band ***Titinopathy should be considered in patient with chronic inflammatory myopathy resistant to treatment
Distal myopathy with rimmed vacuoles (GNE or Nonaka myopathy)	ARD	GNE gene mutation on Ch.9 that encodes GNE protein	• Child or adult onset • Jewish/Arab race • Distal > proximal symmetrical weakness	CK is ↑ EMG: myopathic NCT: non-specific	• Mild variation in fiber size • Could be non-specific • Myopathic change • Minimal focal inflammation • Multiple rimmed vacuoles EM: TFI and myofibrillar disruption

Myopathies with specified or none-specified gene mutations	ADD XLR	1. Zebra body myopathy: ACTA1 gene mutation on Ch.1q42 encodes α-Actin 2. Cap disease: TPM2 gene mutation on Ch.9q13 encodes tropomyosin protein 3. Reducing body myopathy: FHL1 gene mutation on Ch.Xq26 encodes Domain-1,2 protein 4. Spheroid body myopathy: MYOT gene mutation on Ch.5q23 encodes myotilin 5. Fingerprint body myopathy: 6. Cylindrical spiral myopathy: rare EBF3 gene mutation	• Early onset • Generalized weakness • Generalized hypotonia • Spinal rigidity • Scoliosis • Cardiomyopathy • Respiratory failure	CK is normal or ↑ EMG: myopathic NCT: non-specific	• Mild variation in fiber size • Myopathic change • Peripheral caps: purple on H&E, blue on GT, and brown on ATPase- aggregate desmin • Reducing body: granular red in H&E, dark green on GT • Fingerprint inclusion: red in H&E and dark green on GT <u>EM:</u> • Z line fragments/filament (2) • Zebra bodies (1) • Reducing bodies (3) • Fingerprint bodies in (5)
Rippling muscle disease	Immune ADD	Caveolin-3 gene mutation on Ch.3p25.3 encodes caveolin protein. Allelic with LGMD-1C and hypercreatinkinesemia	• Muscle pain and stiffness • Muscle weakness • Toe walking • Muscle contraction • Cardiomyopathy	CK is high EMG: myopathic NCT: non-specific	• Mild variation in muscle size • Selective type II hypertrophy • Multiple internal nuclei • Reduced caveolin stain <u>EM:</u> absent caveolae
Myasthenic syndromes (MGD)	Immune ARD	Autoimmune disease. **Type I:** Myasthenia gravis: IgG antibody to ACH receptor or tyrosine kinase receptor in post synaptic membrane of NMJ **Type II:** Eaton Lambert (ELS): IgG antibody to calcium channel receptor at pre-synaptic membrane of NMJ **Type III:** Neuromyotonia: IgG antibody to potassium channel receptor at pre-synaptic membrane of NMJ **Congenital: many variants. Most common CHAT on Ch. 19q11	• Early or adult onset • Floppy baby • Female > male • Generalized fatigability and weakness increased during day and exercise • Bilateral ptosis • Diplopia • Peripheral neuropathy • Can be associated with dysphagia, respiratory failure, rheumatoid arthritis, lymphoma, diabetes mellitus, BCIM, thymoma • ELS can be associated with cancer or GVHD	High ESR and CRP CK is normal Serology: IgG Ab to ACHR/LRP4 • Tension test • ANA (+) EMG: decrement effect in MGD and increment effect in ELS	• Wild variation in fiber size • Selective type II atrophy • Small angulated fibers • Type I hypertrophy • Multiple internal nuclei • Endomysial fibrosis • Scattered lymphocytes • Rare tubular aggregates

(Continued)

125

Table 17.1 Inherited myopathic diseases not part of muscular dystrophy or other acquired myopathies. *(Continued)*

Disease	Pattern	Cause	Clinical features	Investigation	Microscopic features
Myotonic syndromes	**Type I** ARD **Type II** ADD **Type III** ADD	Delayed relaxation or sustained contractions of skeletal muscle **Type I:** Baker myotonia: due to CLCN1 gene mutation on Ch.7q35 encodes chloride channel receptor **Type II:** Paramyotonia: due to SCN4A gene mutation on Ch.17q23 encodes sodium channel alpha subunit receptor **Type III:** Hyperkalemic periodic paralysis: due to SCN4A or KCNE3 gene mutation on Ch.17q23 encodes sodium and potassium channels	• Early or adult onset • Myotonia • Muscle weakness increases with cold • Distal weakness • Muscle hypertrophy • Flaccid proximal weakness in type III • Dysrhythmia	CK is normal or ↑ EMG: • Myopathic • Myotonia • Fibrillation • Decrement effect Genetic test	• Wide variation in fiber size • Myopathic change • Always non-specific changes • Selective type II hypertrophy • Multiple internal nuclei • Tubular aggregates • Subsarcolemmal vacuoles • Reduced ClC-1 protein stain <u>EM:</u> Tubular aggregates ultrastructural features
Congenital fiber type disproportion (CFTD)	**Type I** ADD **Type II** ARD **Type III** ARD	**Type I:** ACTA1 gene mutation on Ch.1q42 encodes α-actin protein **Type II:** ACTA1 gene mutation on Ch.Xq13 encodes α-actin protein **Type III:** SEPN1 gene mutation on Ch.1p36 encodes selenoprotein-N **Type IV:** TPM3 gene mutation on Ch.1q21 encodes tropomyosin	• Early onset • Adult onset "very rare" • Asymptomatic • Generalized hypotonia • Generalized weakness • Reduced reflexes • Facial weakness • Bulbar symptoms • Scoliosis • Arthrogryposis • Respiratory failure	CK is normal EMG: myopathic	• Minimal variation in fiber size • Type I fiber predominance • Small type I fibers • Large type II fibers • Absent type IIB fibers • Few internal nuclei • Rare nemaline rods on GT

Abbreviations: ADD: autosomal dominant disease. ARD: autosomal recessive, disease. XLD: X-linked disease. RYR-1: ryanodine receptor-1. SR: sarcoplasmic reticulum. SEPN1: selenoprotein-1. ACTA-1: actin alpha-1. NEB: nebulin. TPM2: Tropomyosin beta. MTM1: myotubularin. TTNT1: Troponin-1 isoform. CNM1: centronuclear myoapthy gene. MYOT: myotilin. SLONM: sporadic late-onset nemaline myopathy. DES: desmin. CRYAB: alpha-crystallin B. MYOT: myotilin. ZASP: Z-band spliced PDZ-motif protein. FLNC: filamin-C. BAG3: BCL-2 associated athanogene 3. FHL1: Four and a half LIM domains protein. TTN: titin. STIM1: stromal interaction molecule 1. ORA1: calcium release-activated calcium modulator 1. NMJ: neuromuscular junction. ESR: erythrocyte sedimentation rate. CRP: C-reactive protein. CLCN1: chloride channel protein 1. SCN4A: sodium channel protein type 4 subunit alpha. KCNE3: potassium voltage-gated channel Isk-related family, member 3. EMG: electromyography. NCT: nerve conduction test. CK: creatinine kinase. EM: electron microscopy. GT: Gomori trichrome. HMERF: Hereditary myopathy with early respiratory failure. GNE: UDP-N-acetylglucosamine 2-epimerase/nacetylmannosamine kinase. TFI: tubulofilamentous inclusion. ACH: acetylcholine receptor. BCIM: brachiocephalic inflammatory myopathy. LRP4: lipoprotein receptor-related protein-4. ANA: antinuclear antibody. GVHD: graft versus host disease. MGUS: monoclonal gammopathy of undetermined significance.

multiple central cores or minicores in muscle fibers. These cores are always type I fiber predominant. Pathologists should understand two points: First: the cores should be differentiated from the holes made by freezing artifacts or ice-crystal artifacts; second: not any muscle fiber containing cores means core myopathy. Cores may present in other neuromuscular conditions such as denervation-reinnervation and myofibrillar myopathy (MFM).

The cores seen in CCD express desmin aggregation, devoid of oxidative enzymes, and are best visualized ultrastructurally (**Figure 17.1a–c**). The distinction of structured cores from unstructured cores has no diagnostic significance. In unstructured cores, ATPase activity is lost and there is severe myofibrillar disruption with Z-line streaming (**Figure 17.1c**). Some cases may show multiple centrally positioned nuclei that mimic the diagnosis of

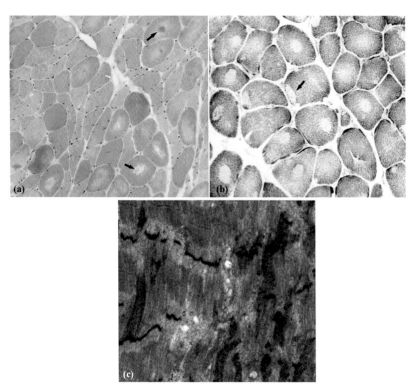

Figure 17.1 Histological sections from a 28-year-old man with core myopathy. **(a)** H&E section shows several muscle fibers with central cores (*black arrows*). **(b)** SDH section shows structural real cores (*black arrow*). *This figure was published in Muscle biopsy: A practical approach, Chapter 15, V. Dubowitz, Congenital myopathies and related disorders, Page 363, Copyright Elsevier 2013.* **(c)** EM ultrastructural section shows unstructured cores with delineated Z-line stream. **(a)** & **(b)** ×25.

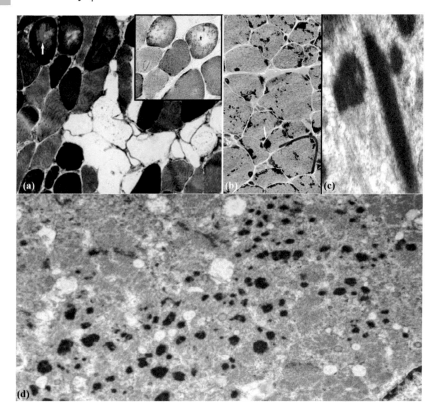

Figure 17.2 (a) NADH and COX sections show multiple minicores (*white arrow,**). **(b)** Gomori trichrome section from 8-year-old boy with severe nemaline rod myopathy (NRM). The rods are seen green-blue in the periphery of the muscle fiber (*white arrow*). **(c, d)** EM section from muscle fibers of a patient with NRM, which shows small electron dense rod-structures. Reprinted with permission from Dr. Robert Hammond, Western University, Canada.

centronuclear myopathy. Genetic analysis can confirm the RYR-1 mutation. Mutations in the C-terminal exons often show the classical central core pathology and account for 66% of cases.

Minicore myopathy (MCM) has similar clinical and histological presentation and genetic abnormalities of CCD. In contrast to central cores, MCM is an autosomal recessive pattern associated with axial weakness, spinal rigidity, more cardiac involvement, and histologically shows small minicores not usually delineated by desmin (**Figure 17.2a**). Pathologists should make careful inspection of muscle fibers with minicores as these cases may sometimes be misdiagnosed with RYR-1 or SEPN1 MCM. They also can be identified in other neuromuscular diseases. (See *Chapter 11, Table 11.1*.)

Nemaline rod structure is a pathological spectrum associated with several neuromuscular diseases. Not every nemaline rod means nemaline rod myopathic disease. Pathologists should be well-oriented about patients' clinical history. **Nemaline rod myopathy** (NRM) is characterized histologically by the presence of multiple small rods in the muscle fibers, which are best visualized by Gomori trichrome stain (GT). Rods are seen green-blue by GT, dark-blue by NADH, and ultrastructurally seen as small elongated electron-dense structures (**Figure 17.2b–d**). The common childhood type of NRM is in the nebulin (NEB) gene mutation on exon 55. Late adult-onset type is observed in cases with ACTA1 gene mutation.

The terms *myotubular myopathy* (MTM) and *centronuclear myopathy* (CNM) share similar histopathological features but different genetic mutations. In **Table 17.1**, we merged these two entities in one category to make it easier for the reader. Both conditions present in early life and are associated with severe systemic illness. Histologically, they present with multiple large central nuclei accompanied with perinuclear halos (**Figure 17.3a**). Female carriers

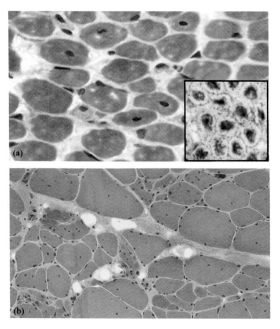

Figure 17.3 Histological sections ×25. **(a)** H&E section from a 4-year-old boy with centronuclear myopathy (CNM) that shows multiple muscle fibers with large central nuclei and rare cytoplasmic bodies and perinuclear halos seen in NADH section. Reprinted with permission from Dr. Robert Hammond, Western University, Canada. **(b)** H&E section from a male patient who presented with titinopathy. There is marked myopathic change with protein aggregates and rimmed vacuoles.

with MTM have shown skewed X-activation. The clinical severity is variable and histologically may show some large central nuclei. Necklace fibers with increased periodic acid-Schiff (PAS) deposition were noted in some carrier cases (**Figure 17.4**). The most common differential diagnosis of CNM or

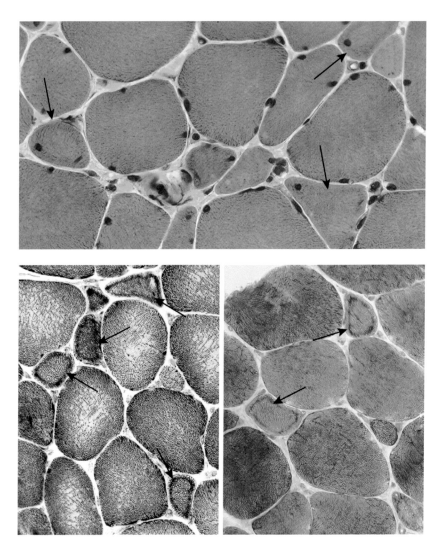

Figure 17.4 Histological sections of different stains show muscle fibers with "nickel place" seen in myotubular myopathy (*black arrow*). This figure was published in Muscle biopsy: A practical approach, Chapter 15, V. Dubowitz, Congenital myopathies and related disorders, Page 382, Copyright Elsevier 2013.

MTM is congenital myotonic dystrophy. Because it is difficult to distinguish these entities histologically, genetic testing is the best standard method.

Titinopathy is an uncommon neuromuscular disease of a mutation in TTN gene. It is allelic and associated with several abnormal variants (**Table 17.1**). It is histologically typical to features seen in MFM (**Figure 17.3b**). The only way to differentiate between these two entities is genetic testing. Titinopathy should also be suspected in cases of inflammatory myopathies when they become nonresponsive to medical therapies.

Myofibrillar myopathy (MFM) is one of the common neuromuscular diseases in muscle pathology with different subsets and variants. The clinical history, genetics, and muscle pathology features are well-described in **Table 17.1**. The histomolecular basis of this group of diseases has now been clearly determined. Because MFM is restricted to conditions in which Z-line proteins are implicated, they share similar pathological features that include abnormal aggregation of several proteins and scattered vacuoles. Most MFMs are sporadic in nature but inheritance pattern can occur as autosomal dominant or recessive. Histopathologically, MFM is characterized by diffuse myopathic features, protein aggregates, and rimmed vacuoles (**Figure 17.5**). Minimal neuropathic change has been observed in many cases. The protein aggregates look eosinophilic in H&E stain but dark-blue on GT and NADH (**Figure 17.5a–b**). These protein aggregates always express desmin stain (**Figure 17.5c**). Some cases also showed wiped-out areas (core-like lesion) in many muscle fibers (**Figure 17.5d**).

The common differential diagnosis of MFM is cytoplasmic body myopathy, titinopathy, reducing body myopathy, and hereditary myopathy with respiratory failure (HMRF). The latter is characterized by sudden onset of muscle weakness, respiratory failure, hypercapnia, and is histologically similar to MFM. Metabolic myopathies due to glycogen depositions should also be ruled out.

Some inherited myopathic diseases may arise either sporadically from a specific gene mutation, as mentioned before, or through unknown gene mutations such as fingerprint body myopathy and cylindrical spiral myopathy. Hence, these histopathological dominant types can be part of other neuromuscular conditions.

Clinically similar to NRM, **cap disease** is histopathologically characterized with cap-like structures in the peripheral edge of muscle fibers. These cap structures express desmin and actin stains. It should be distinguished from tubular aggregates, nemaline rods, and glycogen bodies (**Table 17.1**).

Reducing body myopathy (RBM) can be misdiagnosed with cytoplasmic body and protein aggregate myopathies. However, careful inspection of clinical history and ultrastructural examination of muscle tissue should help in the differential.

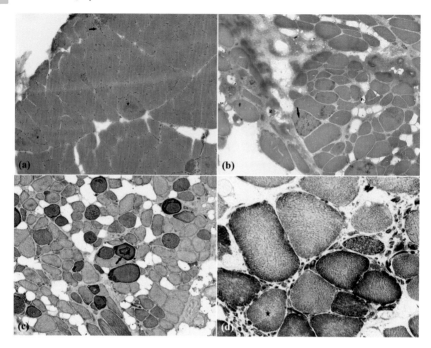

Figure 17.5 Histological sections from a 30-year-old woman with myofibrillar myopathy (desminopathy). **(a)** H&E section shows muscle fibers with eosinophilic aggregates (*) and focal inflammation that mimics titinopathy. **(b)** GT section shows that protein aggregates stain dark blue (*black arrow*). **(c)** Section shows desmin aggregation in many muscle fibers (*black arrow*). **(d)** NADH section shows wiped-out areas in muscle fibers resembling core lesions (*). Different magnifications (×20–×40).

Myotonic syndromes are ion channel disorders characterized by delayed relaxation of skeletal muscles with sustained contraction. It may be accompanied by mild muscle weakness and atrophy. If it becomes worse with exercise, it is called paramyotonia. Myotonic patients present with delayed muscle relaxation such as muscle stiffness and difficult to grip or open eyes. Both myotonia and paramyotonia show characteristic patterns in EMG as a result of repetitive action potentials. This feature unfortunately can be seen in other neuromuscular conditions such as MFM. **Table 17.1** describes the three types of common myotonic syndromes with their genetic variations, clinical presentations, and histopathological differentiation.

One of the common channel disorders in clinical practice is **myasthenia gravis disease** (MGD). It is autoimmune channelopathies due to formation of antibodies against acetylcholine (ACh) receptors. The disease can be diagnosed either clinically through EMG test and Tensilon test or through serological antibody detection against (ACh) or LRP4 (lipoprotein receptor-related protein-4). There are also reports of cases of an autoimmune disorder of caveolin-3 that had antibodies to (ACh-R) and MGD.

Other variants of MGD are Lambert–Eaton syndrome and paramyotonia. These two entities are associated with antibodies against calcium and potassium channel receptors respectively, at a presynaptic membrane of the neuromuscular junction. The whole group of MGDs is histologically unremarkable. They may show some features of selective type II atrophy and rare type I hypertrophy. Anti ACh receptor antibody has also been detected in other neuromuscular conditions such as brachio-cervical myopathy and paraneoplastic syndrome.

Congenital fiber type disproportion (CFTD) is a very rare hereditary disease affecting muscle fiber type distribution. The most common variant is type I, associated with ACTA1 gene mutation. The disease is always early-onset and associated with generalized hypotonia or weakness. It may progress to adulthood. The main pathognomonic sign in muscle biopsy is small type I fibers (40%) versus large type II fibers (60%). There is also a type-I fiber predominance. The diagnosis requires myosin heavy chain stain (slow and fast), to detect muscle fiber type distribution.

In summary, inherited myopathic diseases are characterized pathologically with structural myofibrillar defect, abnormality, or deposition. It should be suspected in early or adult-onset patients presenting with muscle weakness of variable distribution and severity. The gold standard method of diagnosis is muscle biopsy followed by genetic analysis. Genetic counseling of the first-relative degree of the family is important once the mutant gene is newly identified in the patient.

CLINICAL CASE

A 22-year-old man presented to the neuromuscular clinic with slowly progressive and symmetrical weakness and stiffness of proximal muscles at lower limbs for 5 years. He was born a full-term baby with no obstetric complications. No past medical or family history is observed. He has no history of excessive alcohol intake. Neurological examination demonstrates only minimal atrophy of quadriceps muscles with intact reflexes of all limbs. There is no remarkable sensory disturbance.

Serum CK level is elevated (1010 IU/L). EMG of quadriceps muscle shows small brief action potential, indicating mild myopathic pattern. Normal sensory nerve conduction study is observed on NCT.

Based on the Above Findings, What is Your Differential Diagnosis?

A biopsy is done from the left quadriceps muscle. H&E section is illustrated in **Figure 17.6**.

- **Explain the histopathological findings.**
- **What is your likely diagnosis?**

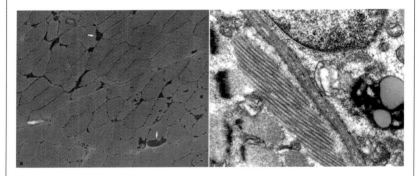

Figure 17.6 Sections from a 22-year-old male show **(a)** muscle fibers with tubular aggregates in H&E stain (*white arrows*). **(b)** EM section shows oblique tubulated structures with honeycomb pattern. Reprinted with permission from Dr. Robert Hammond, Western University, Canada.

Interpretation

H&E section shows minimal myopathic features in the form of scattered atrophic fibers. There are multiple muscle fibers with subsarcolemmal basophilic aggregations, mainly at the periphery of each muscle fiber

(**Figure 17.6a**). These aggregations are red-green on GT stain and dark-blue on NADH stain. There is no COX-SDH negative fibers.

This histological feature is consistent with tubular aggregates. EM sections are performed. Ultrastructurally, there are oblique tubulated structures with honeycomb appearance (**Figure 17.6b**).

These features can be identified in different neuromuscular conditions such as tubular aggregate myopathy (TAM), Limb-girdle myasthenia gravis, exercised-myalgia, hyperkalemic or hypokalemic periodic paralysis, and Stormorken syndrome. Genetic testing is done and revealed STIM1 gene mutation, consistent with TAM.

References

Afifi AK, Smith JW, Zellweger H. Congenital nonprogressive myopathy. Central core and nemaline myopathy in one family. Neurology. 1965; 15: 371–381.

Anderson SL, Ekstein J, Donnelly MC. Nemaline myopathy in the Ashkenazi Jewish population is caused by a deletion in the nebulin gene. Hum Genet. 2004; 115: 185–190.

Argov Z, Eisenberg I, Grabov-Nardini G, et al. Hereditary inclusion body myopathy: the Middle Eastern genetic cluster. Neurology. 2003; 60: 1519–1523.

Bitoun M, Bevilacqua JA, Prudhon B, et al. Dynamin 2 mutations cause sporadic centronuclear myopathy with neonatal onset. Ann Neurol. 2007; 62: 666–670.

Bradley WG, Price DL, Watanabe CK. Familial centronuclear myopathy. J. Neurol Neurosurg Psychiat.1970; 33: 687–693.

Brooke MH, Neville HE. Reducing body myopathy. Neurology. 1972; 22: 829–840.

Chahin N, Selcen D, Engel AG. Sporadic late onset nemaline myopathy. Neurology. 2005; 65: 1158–1164.

Chevessier F, Bauche-Godard S, Leroy JP, et al. The origin of tubular aggregates in human myopathies. J Pathol. 2005; 207: 313–323.

Chinnery PF, Johnson MA, Walls TJ, et al. A novel autosomal dominant distal myopathy with early respiratory failure: clinico-pathologic characteristics and exclusion of linkage to candidate genetic loci. Ann Neurol. 2001; 49: 443–452.

Clarke N. Congenital fiber-type disproportion. Semin Pediatr Neurol. 2011; 18(4): 264–271.

Clarke NF, Domazetovska A, Waddell L, Kornberg A, et al. Cap disease due to mutation of the beta-tropomyosin gene (TPM2). Neuromuscul Disord. 2009; 19: 348–351.

Curless RG, Payne CM, Brinner FM. Fingerprint myopathy: a report of twins. Dev Med Child Neurol. 1978; 20: 793–798.

Dahl N, Hu LJ, Chery M. Myotubular myopathy in a girl with a deletion at Xq27q28 and unbalanced X inactivation assigns the MTM1 gene to a 600-kb region. Am J Hum Genet. 1995; 56: 1108–1115.

Davies NP, Hanna MG. The skeletal muscle channelopathies: basic science, clinical genetics and treatment. Curr Opin Neurol. 2001; 14: 539–551.

Duff RM, Tay V, Hackman P, et al. Mutations in the N-terminal actin-binding domain of filamin C cause a distal myopathy. Am J Hum Genet. 2011; 88: 729–740.

Engel WK, Foster JM, Hughes BP. Central core disease—an investigation of a rare muscle cell abnormality. Brain. 1961; 84: 167–185.

Forrest KM, Al-Sarraj S, Sewry C, et al. Infantile onset myofibrillar myopathy due to recessive CRYAB mutations. Neuromuscul Disord. 2011; 21: 37–40.

Goebel HH, Schloon H, Lenard HG. Congenital myopathy with cytoplasmic bodies. Neuropediatrics. 1981; 12: 166–180.

Helliwell TR, Ellis IH, Appleton RE. Myotubular myopathy: morphological, immunohistochemical and clinical variation. Neuromuscul Disord. 1998; 8: 152–161.

Jungbluth H, Muller CR, Halliger-Keller B, et al. Autosomal recessive inheritance of RYR1 mutations in a congenital myopathy with cores. Neurology. 2002; 59: 284–287.

Martin, JJ, Ceuterick C, Van Goethem G. On a dominantly inherited myopathy with tubular aggregates. Neuromusc Disord. 1997; 7: 512–520.

Ohlsson M, Hedberg C, Bradvik B, et al. Hereditary myopathy with early respiratory failure associated with a mutation in A-band titin. Brain. 2012; 135: 1682–1694.

Reimann J, Kunz WS, Vielhaber S, et al. Mitochondrial dysfunction in myofibrillar myopathy. Neuropathol Appl Neurobiol. 2003; 29: 45–51.

Romero NB, Bevilacqua JA, Oldfors A, et al. Sporadic centronuclear myopathy with muscle pseudohypertrophy, neutropenia, and necklace fibres due to a DNM2 mutation. Neuromuscul Disord. 2011; 21: 148.

Sanoudou D, Beggs AH. Clinical and genetic heterogeneity in nemaline myopathy: a disease of skeletal muscle thin filaments. Trends Mol Med. 2001; 7(8): 362–368.

Sasaki T, Shikura K, Sugai K. Muscle histochemistry in myotubular (centronuclear) myopathy. Brain Dev. 1998; 11: 26–32.

Schessl J, Feldkirchner S, Kubny C, et al. Reducing body myopathy and other FHL1-related muscular disorders. Semin Pediatr Neurol. 2011; 18: 257–263.

Schoser B, Jacob S, Hilton-Jones D, et al. Immune mediated rippling muscle disease with myasthenia gravis: a report of seven patients with long-term follow-up in two. Neuromuscul Disord. 2009; 19: 223–228.

Selcen D. Myofibrillar myopathies. Neuromuscul Disord. 2011; 21: 161–171.

Tajsharghi H, Ohlsson M, Lindberg C, et al. Congenital myopathy with nemaline rods and cap structures caused by a mutation in the beta-tropomyosin gene (TPM2). Arch Neurol. 2007; 64: 1334–1338.

CHAPTER 18

NON-CONGENITAL ACQUIRED MYOPATHIES

Contents

Once the pathologist rules out inflammatory myositis and other inherited muscle diseases, acquired causes should be taken into consideration. Good clinical information and laboratory investigations assist pathologists to shorten the differential diagnosis. It is very difficult to identify the underlying cause from muscle biopsy alone; inputs from clinicians are very important to avoid misdiagnosis.

Myopathies due to systemic diseases, drug toxicity, and long-standing admission in critical care units are not uncommon acquired conditions in clinical practice. **Table 18.1** summarizes these diseases with their causes, clinical manifestations, and histopathological features.

In general, non-congenital acquired myopathies are subclassified, based on their etiology, into three different types:

1. Chronic disease-induced myopathies
2. Toxic myopathies
3. Critical care illness myopathy

18.1 Chronic Disease-Induced Myopathies

Myopathies due to chronic diseases have been described in association with several endocrine disorders, due to an excess or deficiency of thyroid, glucocorticoid, or growth hormone. The muscle involvement is always an incidental feature or may be discovered by exclusion of other conditions through a sequence of laboratory investigations. Pathologists should not

Table 18.1 Non-congenital acquired myopathies.

Disease	Cause	Clinical features	Investigation	Microscopic features
Disease-induced myopathy	1. Endocrine diseases: • Hypothyroidism • Thyrotoxicosis • Cushing's disease • Acromegaly 2. Lymphocytic diseases	• Muscle weakness and pain • Muscle cramps • Fatigability • Myoedema • Peripheral neuropathy • Muscle hypertrophy • Systemic features of each represented disease	CK is ↑ EMG: myopathic NCT: variable	**Hypothyroidism:** • Type I fiber predominance • Fibers with core-like lesion • Glycogen deposition on PAS **Thyrotoxicosis** • Tubular aggregates • Type II atrophy **Cushing's disease:** • Selective type II atrophy • Myosin loss **Acromegaly:** • Segmental necrotic myopathy • Type II atrophy and type I hypertrophy • Enlarged prominent nuclei • Glycogen deposition on PAS **Lymphocytic disease:** • Lymphomyositis: (+) CD4/CD3/MHC class-I

| Toxic myopathy | **Type I:** Focal traumatic myopathy due to intramuscular injection or snake bite **Type II:** Drug-induced myopathy: 1. Ethanol: myonecrosis 2. Steroid: muscle protein loss 3. Statin/fibrate: HMGCoR antibody 4. Cyclosporine: myonecrosis 5. α-Interferon: inflammation 6. Thiazide: hypokalemia 7. AZT: mitochondrial dysfunction 8. Colchicine: lysosomal inhibition 9. Chloroquine: autophagy inhibition 10. Amiodarone: channel blocker 11. Vincristine: microtubule defect | **Clinical staging** • Acute: rhabdomyolysis • Subacute: Painful weakness • Chronic: Painless weakness **Others:** • Peripheral neuropathy • Cardiomyopathy • Retinopathy • Skin rash Note: Rhabdomyolysis is acute non-inflammatory necrotizing myopathy | CK is ↑ AST/ALT ↑ Myoglobinuria EMG: myopathic HMG-CoR AB + in statin myopathy | **Type I:** focal inflammation + necrosis + fibrosis **Type II** • Necrotizing myopathy in **1/3/4/7** • Type II atrophy in **1/2/4** • Inflammatory myopathy in **3/5** • Vacuolar myopathy in **6/8/9/10** • Neuromyopathy in **7/8/9/10/11** • Mitochondrial myopathy in **4/7** • Tubular aggregate in **1/6** • Myosin heavy chain loss in **2** • MHC class-I up-regulation in **3** EM: • Curvilinear bodies in **9** • Tubuloreticular inclusion in **7** |

(Continued)

139

Table 18.1 Non-congenital acquired myopathies. (Continued)

Disease	Cause	Clinical features	Investigation	Microscopic features
Critical care myopathy (CCM)	Long-term dependency of critical ill patient on intensive care unit. **Associated with intravenous injection of high dose of steroid in patient under neuromuscular blockage such as in MGD, sepsis, renal failure, and organs failure	• Painful quadriplegia • Symmetrical distal weakness • Peripheral neuropathy • Areflexia • Respiratory failure	CK is normal or ↑ EMG: myopathic NCT: • Small amplitude • Long duration	• Neuromyopathic change • Loss of H&E stain in some fibers • Selective type II atrophy • Scattered angulated fibers • Regenerated fibers • Central myosin loss • Type I fibers darker in MHCs >MHCf EM: Loss of A-band

Abbreviations: EMG: electromyography. NCT: nerve conduction test. CK: creatinine kinase. EM: electron microscopy. MHC: major histocompatibility. AST: aspartate aminotransferase. ALT: alanine aminotransferase. IMPP: immune myopathy with perimysial pathology. HMGCoR: 3-hydroxy-3-methylglutaryl-coenzyme. AZT: azidothymidine. MGD: myasthenia gravis disease. PAS: periodic acid-Schiff. MHCf: myosin heavy chain-fast. MHCs: myosin heavy chain-slow.

neglect these chronic diseases during muscle biopsy interpretation. The muscle weakness in these disorders can be proportionate to the degree of hormonal deficiency. However, patients become symptomatic when there is a severe hormonal deficiency or toxicity. Many reported studies in the literature reveal minimal non-specific myopathic changes.

Hypothyroid myopathy shows non-specific histological change such as type I fiber predominance, mitochondrial dysfunction, and rare glycogens deposition. *Cushing syndrome-induced myopathy* is commonly associated with selective type II atrophy. This histological feature has also been described in patients with steroid myopathy and paraneoplastic myopathy due to malignancy. Excess growth hormone (*acromegaly*) in adulthood rarely causes myopathy and if so, it may present with alternative features of atrophic and hypertrophic fibers with focal segmental necrosis. Cases with lymphoma reach the myopathic stage when the lymphocytes infiltrate through the muscle. It may mimic granulomatous myositis. T-cell lymphoma is the most common lymphoma affecting the muscle and the lymphocytes expressing CD4, CD68, and MHC class-I.

18.2 Toxic Myopathies

Myotoxicity from drugs or toxins may occur due to several mechanisms, including direct injury to muscle sarcolemma or affecting sarcolemmal proteins via specific immunopathological processes. Although drug-induced myopathies are uncommon, few cases have been reported in the literature with unique myopathological change. Clinical presentations range from focal weakness due to localized effects to painful proximal myopathy or necrotizing myopathy, to painless muscle weakness. The progression of the disease is usually slow and rarely ends with complete loss of muscle power. Some drugs may produce characteristic histological features in muscle biopsy or electron microscopy. The most common drugs causing myopathy in clinical practice are statin, steroid, hydroxychloroquine, colchicine, and zidovudine.

18.2.1 Statin-Induced Myopathy

Statin-induced myopathy is a fairly common condition in clinical practice. Its treatment requires careful attention and close follow-up. The drug is used for the treatment of dyslipidemia with high low-density lipoprotein (LDL) and cholesterol level.

Statins are inhibitors for HMG-CoA reductase, an enzyme that catalyzes the conversion of HMG-CoA to mevalonic acid, the precursor of cholesterol. They lower the cholesterol and LDL levels in the blood. They could interrupt cholesterol metabolism causing damage to the muscle sarcolemma and mitochondria, allowing the influx of calcium to the cells resulting in myonecrosis.

The myotoxicity associated with statin affects 1%–7% of all patients taking the medication; this toxicity is greatly increased by co-administration of other cholesterol-lowering agents, such as fenofibrate.

Patients taking statin may suffer from mild muscle cramps, particularly at night. This cramp usually gets worse during physical exercise. It may progress slowly to cause symmetrical muscle weakness or rarely an acute rhabdomyolysis. The CK level is rarely elevated above 1000 IU/L. Some evidence suggests that the toxicity is dose-related, but that was from general meta-analyses. If the patient starts to have a high CK level above 10,000 with progressive muscle weakness and pain, statin-induced myopathy should be suspected in patients taking statin.

Detection of HMGCoR reductase antibody through ELISSA is a newly developed test used to confirm the diagnosis of immune-mediated necrotizing myopathy. However, muscle biopsy is strongly indicated to rule out other inflammatory myopathies.

Statin-induced myopathy can present histopathologically by one of the following syndromes:

- *Immune-mediated necrotizing myopathy*: It is characterized by scattered necrotic fibers, minimal histiocytic inflammation, and MHC Class-I upregulation in non-necrotic fibers. Perimysial fragmentation might be seen. This spectrum is histologically close to immune-myopathy with perimysial pathology.
- *Inflammatory myositis*: Some reported cases, treated with simvastatin and atorvastatin, were found to have dermatomyositis. It is histologically characterized by focal inflammation, regenerated muscle fibers, and focal perifascicular atrophy.

18.3 Critical Care Illness Myopathy

This rare spectrum often occurs due to long-term dependency of the patient in a critical care unit. It can be aggregated by intravenous injection of high doses of steroid under neuromuscular blockage and mechanical ventilation. Muscle biopsy shows minimal neuromyopathic features, type II fiber atrophy, and myosin change (**Table 18.1**).

CLINICAL CASE

A 51-year-old woman presented to the neurology clinic with gradual pain and weakness of quadriceps muscle for 2 months. She has a known history of controlled diabetes, hypertension, dyslipidemia, gout, and rheumatoid arthritis. She drinks alcohol occasionally. She denies any bulbar symptoms, ophthalmoplegia, and rash. The patient is on multiple medications include statin, allopurinol, hydroxychloroquine, amlodipine, and metformin. Neurological examination is unremarkable. There is no remarkable sensory disturbance.

Serum CK level is highly elevated (8900 IU/L). ANA test is positive. EMG shows minimal myopathic pattern. Normal sensory nerve conduction study is observed on NCT.

Based on the Above Findings, What is Your Differential Diagnosis?

A biopsy is done from her right quadriceps muscle. Histological sections are illustrated in **Figure 18.1**.

- **Explain the histopathological findings.**
- **What is your likely diagnosis?**

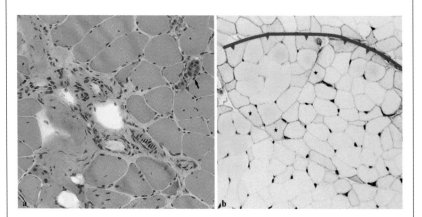

Figure 18.1 Histological sections from a 51-year-old woman with statin-induced necrotizing myopathy. **(a)** H&E section shows myopathic features with phagocytosed necrotic fiber (*black arrow*). **(b)** MHC class-I upregulation in non-necrotic muscle fibers (*).×20.

Interpretation

H&E section shows severe necrotizing myopathy with focal histiocytic inflammation. No cytological inclusions are found. Some regenerated fibers are identified (**Figure 18.1a**). MHC class-I is expressed in some non-necrotic muscle fibers with minimal upregulation in vasculature (**Figure 18.1b**). This histological feature is consistent with the diagnosis of immune-mediated necrotizing myopathy. This is commonly associated with statin-induced Myopathy.

References

Afifi AK, Bergman RA, Harvey JC. Steroid myopathy. Clinical, histologic and cytologic observations. Johns Hopkins Med J. 1968; 123: 158–173.

Beil M, Chariot P. Muscle disorders associated with cyclosporine treatment. Muscle Nerve. 1999; 22(12): 1631–1636.

Bischoff A, Esslen E. Myopathy with primary hyperparathyroidism. Neurology. 1965; 15: 64–68.

Carvalho AA, Lima UW, Valiente RA. Statin and fibrate associated myopathy: study of eight patients. Arq Neuropsiquiatr. 2004; 62: 257–261.

Dalakas MC. Toxic and drug-induced myopathies. J Neurol Neurosurg Psychiatry. 2009; 80: 832–838.

Darnell RB, Posner JB. Paraneoplastic syndromes involving the nervous system. N Engl J Med. 2003; 349: 1543–1554.

Evans M, Rees A. Effects of HMG-CoA reductase inhibitors on skeletal muscle: are all statins the same? Drug Saf. 2002; 25: 649–663.

Fernandez C, Figarella-Branger D, Alla P, et al. Colchicine myopathy: a vacuolar myopathy with selective type I muscle fiber involvement. An immunohistochemical and electron microscopic study of two cases. Acta Neuropathol. 2002; 103(2): 100–106.

Grable-Esposito P, Katzberg HD, Greenberg AR, et al. Immune-mediated necrotizing myopathy associated with statins. Muscle Nerve. 2010; 41(2): 185–190.

Kawaguchi N, Izumi R, Kobayashi M, et al. Extranodal NK/T-cell lymphoma mimicking granulomatous myositis. Intern Med. 2019; 58(2): 277–282.

Lacomis D, Zochodne DW, Bird SJ. Critical illness myopathy. Muscle Nerve 2000; 23(12): 1785–1788.

Lane RJM, McLean KA, Moss J, et al. Myopathy in HIV infection: the role of zidovudine and the significance of tubuloreticular inclusions. Neuropathol Appl Neurobiol. 1993; 19: 406–413.

Lin RT, Liu CK, Tai CT, Lai CL. Hypothyroid myopathy-pathological and ultrastructural study. Kaohsiung J Med Sci. 2000; 16(2): 68–75.

Mastaglia FL. Pathological changes in skeletal muscle in acromegaly. Acta Neuropathol. 1973; 24: 273–286.

Müller R, Kugelberg E. Myopathy in Cushing's syndrome. J Neurol Neurosur Psychiatry. 1995; 22: 314–319.

Needham M, Fabian V, Knezevic W, et al. Progressive myopathy with up-regulation of MHC-I associated with statin therapy. Neuromuscul Disord. 2003; 17: 194–200.

Oztas M, Ugurlu S, Aydin O. Atorvastatin-induced dermatomyositis. Rheumatol It. 2017; 37(7): 1217–1219.

Simon L, Jolley SE, Molina PE. Alcoholic myopathy: pathophysiologic mechanisms and clinical implication. Alcohol Res. 2017; 38(2): 2017–2217.

CHAPTER 19

METABOLIC MYOPATHY

Contents

Metabolic myopathy is a diverse group of rare genetic disorders characterized by abnormal accumulation of proteins or metabolic products in muscle fibers. Impairments of glycolysis, glycogenolysis, fatty acid oxidation, or mitochondrial respiratory chains represent the majority of the accumulated products. These materials are aggregated in a group of vacuoles, referred to as *vacuolar myopathy*. The approach was explained in detail in *Chapter 15*.

Patients with metabolic disease initially present with subtle myopathic features and exercise intolerance. It can occur at any age, but early-childhood onset presents with generalized hypotonia "floppy baby syndrome." Late-adulthood presentation was commonly reported in the literature and usually associated with systemic organ diseases. The clinician needs a strong suspicion to distinguish the metabolic diseases from other conditions with similar presentations. Laboratory tests always show non-specific results. However, abnormal liver enzymes and glucose disturbance may occur in severe conditions.

Targeted enzyme activity measurement using tandem spectroscopy (TS) as well as next-generation sequencing (NGS) is increasingly used. This molecular testing is not usually done until muscle biopsy rules out other common abnormal neuromuscular conditions.

Any muscle biopsy showing non-inflammatory necrotizing myopathy in young patients should raise the suspicion of metabolic myopathies. The biopsy is generally characterized by moderate-to-severe necrotizing myopathy with or without vacuolations. The vacuolation contains solid eosinophilic materials and is associated with variable staining patterns based on the underlying metabolic abnormality.

Because these disorders are treatable, specific enzyme-replacement therapies are now available, and other metabolic strategies and gene therapies are undergoing clinical trials.

Metabolic myopathies can be subclassified into the following groups:

1. Glycogen storage diseases
2. Lipid storage diseases
3. Mitochondrial myopathies
4. Others: such as polyglucosan body disease, myoadenylate deaminase deficiency, and amyloid myopathy.

Table 19.1 summarizes the genetic definition, clinical presentation, and histopathological features of metabolic myopathies.

19.1 Glycogen Storage Diseases (GSD, Glycogenosis)

Any minor defect in the glycolytic pathway will cause fatigue, muscle cramps, or rhabdomyolysis, which are considered essential signs for glycogenosis. The main underlying pathology is glycogen deposition in several organs including skeletal muscles. The inheritance of these disorders is usually autosomal recessive. Histologically, the muscle shows scattered degenerated and necrotic fibers with subsarcolemmal and central vacuolations containing solid materials. These materials are glycogen droplets, and their types are dependent on the specific deficient enzyme (Figure 19.1). The most common type is glycogenosis type-II (Pompe disease). Other glycogen storage diseases are summarized in Table 19.1.

19.1.1 Pompe Disease

Pompe disease is the most common glycogen storage disease in clinical practice that is characterized clinically by spinal muscular atrophy-like disease, floppy baby syndrome, and facial dysmorphism. Patients can also present in late adulthood with variable weakness distribution ranging from proximal weakness to limb-girdle muscular weakness. The disease may progress to involve organs such as liver, spleen, lungs, and, rarely, heart. The disease is inherited as autosomal recessive and associated with GAA gene mutation, which causes deficiency of acid maltase or α-1, 4-glycosidase enzyme.

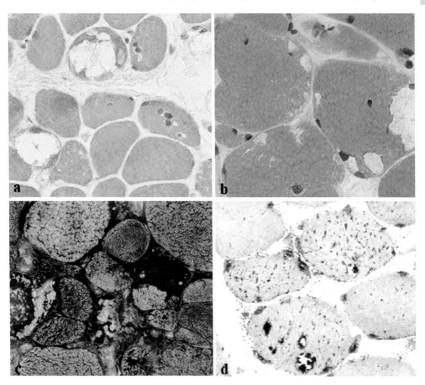

Figure 19.1 Histological sections of muscle tissue from patients with glycogen storage diseases. **(a)** Pompe disease with sarcoplasmic vacuoles containing glycogen. **(b)** Cori Forbes disease with large subsarcoplasmic vacuoles with glycogen deposition. **(c)** PAS stain reveals excessive glycogen depositions in the muscle fibers. **(d)** Increased acid phosphatase activity in the vacuoles of patients with Pompe disease. Reprinted with permission from Dr. Robert Hammond, Western University, Canada. ×25.

When you suspect Pompe disease, send the dried blood test on a filter paper for tandem spectroscopy to detect enzyme deficiency. The muscle biopsy and dried blood test should be done in the same time. However, NGS is considered the best confirmatory method for the diagnosis.

Muscle biopsy shows pure myopathic features with scattered atrophic, necrotic, and regenerated fibers. The most striking feature is the presence of central and subsarcolemmal vacuolations containing glycogens, stained pink-red with PAS stain (**Figure 19.1a, c**). The glycogen is digested by PAS-diastase. The enzyme is present in the lysosome and there is consequently

Table 19.1 Classification of metabolic myopathies.

Disease	Pattern	Cause	Clinical features	Investigation	Microscopic features
Glycogen storage diseases (Glycogenosis)	ARD	**Type 0:** GYS-1 gene mutation on Ch.19q13 causes glycogen synthetase enzyme deficiency. **Type II:** Pompe disease: GAA gene mutation on Ch.17q25 causes α-1, 4-glycosidase "acid maltase" enzyme deficiency. Allelic with LGMD 2V. **Type III:** Cori Forbes disease: AGL gene mutation on Ch.1p21 causes amylo1, 6-glycosidase deficiency. **Type IV:** Amylopectinosis/ Andersen's disease: GBE1 gene mutation on Ch.3p12 causes 1,4 α-glucan branching deficiency. **Type V:** McArdle disease: PYGM gene mutation on Ch.11q13 causes phosphorylase deficiency. **Type VII:** Tarui's disease: PFKM gene mutation on Ch.12q13 causes 6-phosphofructokinase deficiency. **Type IX:** PGK1 gene mutation on Ch.Xq21 that causes phosphoglycerate kinase deficiency. **Type X:** PGAM-2 gene mutation on Ch.7p13 that can cause phosphoglycerate mutase deficiency. **Type XI:** LDHA gene mutation on Ch.11p15 causes lactate dehydrogenase deficiency	• Early or adult onset • Male>female • Italian and Jewish • Easy fatigability • Exertional cramp • Generalized weakness **Type II:** • Floppy baby syndrome • Facial dysmorphism • Cardiomyopathy • Hepatosplenomegaly • Calf hypertrophy • Scapular winging • LGMD weakness • Contractures • Can be associated with hydrocephalus **Type V:** • Muscle wasting • Renal failure • Myoglobinuria • High risk to MH **Type VII/IX** associated with hemolytic anemia	• CK is normal or ↑ • Hyperkalemia Hypoglycemia • Myoglobinuria • Hyperuricemia • Liver enzymes ↑ • GAA activity • PFK activity • EMG: myopathic with fibrillation and myotonia • Skin fibroblast • Gene seq. **Others to do:** ECG Echocardiograph	• Wide variation in fiber size • Necrosis and regeneration • Multiple internal nuclei **Type 0:** • Diffuse glycogen depletion • Many fibers with (-) PAS • Type I fiber predominance **Type II:** • Subsarcolemmal vacuolation containing glycogen deposits (+) PAS and cleared with PAS-D • (+) Acid PO4 activity in vacuoles • Autophagic vacuoles stained by spectrin • MCH class I up-regulation **Type V:** • Subsarcolemmal vacuolation containing glycogen deposits (+) PAS • Fiber linearization on NADH • Rimmed vacuoles • Absent phosphorylase stain except in regenerating fibers **Type VII and X:** • Subsarcolemmal vacuolation containing glycogen deposits (+) PAS • Tubular aggregate in **type X** EM: • Myofibrillar disruption • Membrane-bound glycogen • Autophagic vacuoles • Abnormal mitochondrial proliferation
Glycogen storage disease with normal acid maltase (Danon disease)	XLD	LAMP-2 gene nonsense mutation on Ch.Xq24 encodes laminin α-2. **Allelic with SPMD	• Muscle weakness • Hypoglycemia • Hepatomegaly • Mental retardation • Cardiomyopathy	• CK is ↑↑ • EMG: myopathic • Glucose is low • Ketone is low	• Myopathic change • Subsarcolemmal vacuoles containing glycogen droplets (+) PAS but (-) for acid PO4 activity • Lectin labeling in vacuoles • Absent laminin α-2

Lipid storage diseases (LSD)	ARD	Fatty acid-B-oxidation defect **Type I:** Carnitine deficiency due to OCTN2 (SLC22A5) gene mutation on Ch.5q31 encoded carnitine **Type II:** Carnitine palmitoyl-transferase II deficiency due to CPT2 mutation on Ch.1p32 **Type III:** Acyl-CoA dehydrogenase deficiency due to different gene mutations (ACADS, ACDM, ACADVL, ETF)	• Infantile or adult onset • Generalized cramps • Muscle weakness • Weight loss • Recurrent myoglobinuria • Cardiomyopathy • Encephalopathy (type I) • Hepatomegaly • Hypoglycemia • Can be associated with Fanconi syndrome	CK is ↑ Lactate is ↑ Ammonia is ↑ Glucose is low Ketone is low EMG: myopathic Gene seq.	• Mild variation in fiber size • Non-specific change • Type II muscle atrophy • Vacuoles with lipid deposition seen more in type I fibers, red/brown with oil-red and black with Sudan black • Absent glycogen on PAS stain • Punctate cytoplasm • Autophagic vacuoles EM: Excessive lipid droplets and abnormal mitochondrial aggregation
Polyglucosan body myopathy (PGBM)	ARD	**Type I:** RBCK1 gene mutation on Ch.20p13 encodes E3-ubiquitin ligase **Type II:** GYG-1 gene mutation on Ch.3q24 encodes glycogenin protein	• Child onset • Proximal weakness • Ptosis • Cardiomyopathy • Hepatomegaly • Immunodeficiency	CK is normal or ↑ Serum IgA ↑ EMG: myopathic ECG	• Mild variation in fiber size • Diffuse glycogen depletion • Polyglucosan body (+) for ubiquitin, P-62 and PAS but PAS-D resistant • Desmin aggregation
Myoadenylate deaminase deficiency (MADD)	ARD	AMPD-1 gene mutation on Ch.1p13 causes myoadenylate deaminase enzyme deficiency Low ATP production	• Fatigability • Muscle pain • Muscle weakness	Lactate is normal Low AMP: normal	• Myopathic changes • Scattered necrotic fibers • Tubular aggregates • Absent AMPD stain in fibers

Mitochondria myopathies	Sporadic	Maternal inheritance of heteroplasmic mitochondrial DNA or rRNA gene mutations. **Variants associated with myopathies are:**
		  I. MELAS
		  II. MERRF
		  III. CPEO
		  IV. MNGIE
		  V. Isolated myopathy
		  VI. NARP
		Secondary causes: See *Table 11.1*
			• Muscle weakness
			• Bilateral ptosis
			• External opthalmoplegia
			• SNHL
			• Myoclonic epilepsy
			• Sideroblastic anemia
			• Brain calcifications
			• Cardiomyopathy
				CK is ↑ or N
				Lactate is ↑
				Brain MRI
				Gene seq.
					• Wide variation in fiber size
					• Rare necrotic and regenerated fibers
					• Subsarcolemmal basophilia seen as ragged-red fibers (RRF) on GT and ragged-blue fibers (RBF) on SDH and NADH stain
					• Scattered COX (–) fibers
					• Scattered fibers with large lipid droplets
					*EM: Myofibrillar disruption
					Crystalline/paracrystalline inclusions
					Mitochondrial proliferation
					Swollen SR

(Continued)

Table 19.1 Classification of metabolic myopathies. (Continued)

Disease	Pattern	Cause	Clinical features	Investigation	Microscopic features
Amyloid myopathy	Acquired Inherited ADD	A. **Primary**: hereditary Transthyretin related FAP: **Type I/II**: TTR gene mutation (Val30met) on Ch.18q12 **Type III**: APOA1 gene mutation on Ch.11q23 **Type IV**: GSN gene mutation on Ch. 9q33 B. **Secondary**: acquired causes: chronic infection, SLE, RA, and Polyarteritis nodosa	• Usually asymptomatic • Adult onset • Common in Portuguese • Proximal > distal muscle weakness and pain • Peripheral neuropathy • Autonomic dysfunction • Carpal tunnel syndrome • Dysphagia • Weight loss • Cardiomyopathy	CK is normal EMG: myopathic NCT: neuropathic	• Mild variation in muscle size • Rare necrotic fibers • Denervation change • Amyloid deposition (PV/PM) stained + for Congo red and TTR labeling • Autophagic vacuoles • Axonal neuropathy EM: amyloid fibrils (8-15 nm) Autophagic vacuoles—segmental demyelination

Abbreviations: ADD: autosomal dominant disease. ARD: autosomal recessive disease. XLD: X-linked disease. EMG: electromyography. NCT: nerve conduction test. CK: creatinine kinase. N: normal. MRI: magnetic resonance imaging. EM: electron microscopy. GT: Gomori trichrome stain. GYS: glycogen synthetase enzyme deficiency. OCTN: organic cationic transporter. CPT2: Carnitine palmitoyl-transferase II. ACAD: acyl CoA dehydrogenase. ETF: electron transfer flavoprotein. SNHL: Sensioneuronal hearing loss. MELAS: myopathy-encephalopathy-lactic acidosis and stroke-like episodes. MERRF: myoclonic epilepsy with ragged red fibers. CPEO: chronic progressive external ophthalmoplegia. MNGIE: mitochondrial gastrointestinal encephalopathy. SR: sarcoplasmic reticulum. NARP: neuropathy, ataxia, retinitis pigmentosa. MH: malignant hyperthermia. PFK: phosphofructokinase. ECG: echocardiogram. PAS: periodic acid-Schiff. PAS-D: periodic acid Schiff-diastase. GAA: glycosidase enzyme activity. AGL: amylo 1,5-glycosidase enzyme. PYGM: glycogen phosphorylase muscle associated. PFKM: phosphofructokinase muscle. PGK1: phosphoglycerate kinase. LDH1: lactate dehydrogenase. GYG-1: glycogenin-1. SPMD: scapuloperoneal muscular dystrophy. FAP: familial amyloid polyneuropathy. TTR: transthyretin. APOA1: apolipoprotein-1. GSN: gelsolin. SLE: systemic lupus erythematosus. RA: rheumatoid arthritis. PV: perivascular. PM: perimysial. AMPD: myoadenylate deaminase.

abundance in acid phosphatase activity (**Figure 19.1d**). There is also MHC class-I upregulation in most muscle fibers, of undetermined significance.

One of the common differential diagnoses of Pompe disease is Danon disease, type-III GSD and GSD-V. Danon disease is an x-linked pattern characterized by subsarcolemmal vacuolations of glycogen droplets but with normal acid maltase enzyme and no acid phosphatase activity in the vacuoles. Labeling of lectin in the vacuoles was shown in Danon disease but not in Pompe disease.

McArdle disease is a type-V glycogen storage disease that commonly occurs in young patients with recurrent myoglobinuria and exertional cramps. The vacuoles are very fine and smaller than the ones described in Pompe disease. It is associated with absent phosphorylase enzymes in muscle fibers.

The histological picture of Cori Forbes disease is very similar to Pompe disease. However, the vacuoles are more tinged, large, and diffuse to involve most muscle fibers (**Figure 19.1b**).

Complete absence of glycogen in muscle fibers is rare and seen in G0 type of glycogen storage disease, due to the GYS-1 gene mutation.

19.2 Lipid Storage Diseases

This spectrum of disorders is very rare. It occurs due to fatty acid beta oxidation defect across the mitochondrial membrane, which leads to abnormal accumulation of lipids in the systemic organs. Although muscle biopsy always demonstrates non-specific change, some cases show vacuoles containing large lipid droplets, commonly seen in type I fibers more than type II fibers. These lipids turn the whole muscle fiber into red/brown with oil-red stain or black with Sudan black stain. The most common underlying cause of this condition is carnitine deficiency (**Table 19.1**). The disease should be suspected in a child with recurrent myoglobinuria, hypoglycemia, and cardiomyopathy.

19.3 Mitochondrial Myopathies (MM)

Because mitochondrial dysfunction can be seen as a secondary abnormality in several myopathic diseases, the term *mitochondrial myopathy* should not be used as a separate entity. The clinician should sort out the cause of these mitochondrial abnormalities.

Primary mitochondrial diseases occur due to defects in enzymes encoded by nuclear genes or those of the mitochondrial genome. As described in *Chapter 1,*

Part I, oxidative phosphorylation and respiratory chain complex are the main essential targeted defects in the cycle of mitochondrial function. Disturbance of the mitochondrial genome (MitDNA) in this complex cycle may cause mitochondrial cytopathies. It has been estimated that MitDNA mutations are responsible for approximately 20%–30% of oxidative phosphorylation diseases, but the majority of oxidative phosphorylation diseases with identified gene defects are due to MitDNA mutations. The manifestations caused by this alteration always involve multiple large-scale deletions and/or reduced copy numbers. These mutations are transmitted only from mother to fetus because MitDNA is maternally inherited.

In muscle biopsy, the muscle tissue is either unremarkable or it may show minimal myopathic features with focal mitochondrial dysfunction. The latter is histologically seen as subsarcolemmal basophilia in muscle fibers (**Figure 19.2a**). This basophilic aggregation is visualized as either ragged-red fibers by Gomori trichrome stain or ragged-blue fibers with oxidative stain (SDH and NADH stain) (**Figure 19.2b–d**). A single muscle fiber with ragged red fiber is enough to diagnose mitochondrial myopathy. COX-negative fibers are other specific histological features of mitochondrial myopathy (**Figure 19.2e**). Bear in mind, ragged fibers should be differentiated from necrotizing degenerating fibers accumulating mitochondria. This can be distinguished by electron microscopy (EM). Ultrastructural examination of diseased tissue of mitochondrial dysfunction shows abnormal mitochondrial aggregation, mitochondrial bloating and enlargement, and paracrystallin inclusions (**Figure 12.1d, l**-*Chapter 12*).

In inclusion body myositis (IBM), ragged red fibers and COX-negative fibers are randomly scattered in muscle fibers. This occurs due to MitDNA mutation associated with IBM. On the other hand, COX-negative fibers in dermatomyositis are distributed in a perifascicular pattern (**Figure 19.1f**).

19.4 Other Metabolic Myopathies

Other types of metabolic myopathies are summarized in **Table 19.1**.

19.4.1 Amyloid Myopathy

Amyloid myopathy is an uncommon metabolic disease characterized by abnormal deposition of amyloid proteins in muscle fibers. Patients may present with early peripheral neuropathy followed by myopathy. Widespread

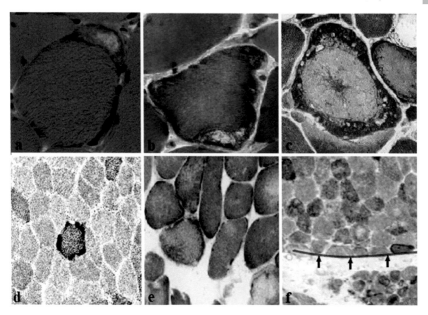

Figure 19.2 Histological sections from a patient with mitochondrial dysfunction (mitochondrial myopathy). **(a)** Subsacrolemmal basophilia on H&E section. **(b)** Ragged-red fiber with Gomori trichrome stain. **(c, d)** Ragged-blue fibers with NADH and SDH stains respectively. **(e)** COX-negative fiber with combined COX-SDH stain. **(f)** Perifascicular COX-negative fibers in dermatomyositis (*black arrows*). This figure was published in Muscle biopsy: A practical approach, Chapter 18, V. Dubowitz, Metabolic myopathies II, Page 477, Copyright Elsevier 2013.

deposition of amyloid may cause systemic amyloidosis that ends with organ damage. The diagnosis is always difficult in clinical ground as amyloidosis is rarely suspected in clinician thoughts. Amyloidosis could be primary due to sporadic or inherited gene mutations or secondary, resulting from underlying chronic illness. A rare example of inherited or sporadic cases is amyloid deposition due to transthyretin. Muscle biopsy demonstrates perivascular and perimysial amyloid deposition. With using EM, the vessels and muscle fibers are lined with elongated and thin amyloid fibrils, frequently seen on the basal lamina.

CLINICAL CASE

A 39-year-old man presented to the neurology clinic with peripheral tingling sensation for 6 months. He recently started to have muscle weakness in the lower limbs and postural hypotension. There is no muscle wasting or calf pseudohypertrophy. The reflexes are intact in neurological examination. General body examination is unremarkable. Serum CK level is normal. EMG/NCT shows minimal myopathic pattern.

Based on the Above Findings, What is Your Differential Diagnosis?

A biopsy is done from his right quadriceps muscle. Histological sections are illustrated in **Figure 19.3a**. EM has also been done (**Figure 19.3b**).

- Explain the histopathological findings.
- What is your likely diagnosis?

Interpretation

H&E section shows evidence of denervation atrophy (**Figure 19.3a**). Because Congo red stains show unremarkable result, EM is performed. Ultrastructural examination of semi-thin sections of muscle tissue shows Perimysial deposition of 15–18 nm amyloid fibrils. The features are consistent with diagnosis of amyloid myopathy.

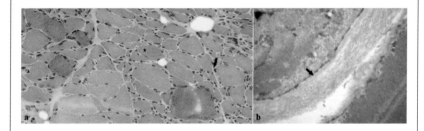

Figure 19.3 Sections from a 39-year-old man with amyloid myopathy. **(a)** H&E section shows denervation atrophy with target fiber (*) and scattered atrophic and angulated fibers (*black arrow*). **(b)** EM thin section shows 15 nm amyloid fibrils surrounding the muscle fiber (*black arrow*).

References

Amendt BA, Greene C, Sweetman L, et al. Short-chain acyl-coenzyme A dehydrogenase deficiency. Clinical and biochemical studies in two patients. J Clin Invest. 1987; 79: 1303–1309.

Anneser JMH, Pongratz DE, Podskarbi T, Shin YS, et al. Mutations in the acid alpha-glucosidase gene (M. Pompe) in a patient with an unusual phenotype. Neurology. 2005; 64: 368–370.

Antonicka H, Sasarman F, Kennaway NG, et al. The molecular basis for tissue specificity of the oxidative phosphorylation deficiencies in patients with mutations in the mitochondrial translation factor EFG1. Hum Mol Genet. 2006; 15: 1835–1846.

Bonnefont JP, Demaugre F, Prip-Buus C, et al. Carnitine palmitoyltransferase deficiencies. Mol Genet Metab. 1999; 68: 424–440.

Bruno C, Cassandrini D, Assereto S, et al. Neuromuscular forms of glycogen branching enzyme deficiency. Acta Myol. 2007. 26: 75–78.

Cameron JM, Levandovskiy V, MacKay N, et al. Identification of a novel mutation in GYS1 (muscle-specific glycogen synthase) resulting in sudden cardiac death, that is diagnosable from skin fibroblasts. Mol Genet Metab. 2005; 98: 378–382.

Chapin JE, Kornfeld M, Harris A. Amyloid myopathy: characteristic features of a still underdiagnosed disease. Muscle Nerve. 2005; 31: 266–272.

Coelho T, Sousa A, Lourenco E, Ramalheira J. A study of 159 Portuguese patients with familial amyloidotic polyneuropathy (FAP) whose parents were both unaffected. J Med Genet. 1994; 31: 293–299.

Danon MJ, Oh SJ, DiMauro S, et al. 1981 Lysosomal glycogen storage disease with normal acid maltase. Neurology. 1981; 31: 51–57.

De Meirleir L, Seneca S, Lissens W, et al. Respiratory chain complex V deficiency due to a mutation in the assembly gene ATP12. J Med Genet. 2004; 41: 120–124.

DiMauro S, Trevisan C, Hays A. Disorders of lipid metabolism in muscle. Muscle Nerve. 1981; 3: 369–388.

Holt IJ, Harding AE, Morgan-Hughes JA. Deletions of muscle mitochondrial DNA in patients with mitochondrial myopathies. Nature. 1988; 331: 717–719.

Illingworth B, Cori GT. Structure of glycogens and amylopectins. III. Normal and abnormal human glycogen. J Biol Chem. 1952; 199: 653–660.

Klein CJ, Boes CJ, Chapin JE, et al. Adult polyglucosan body disease: case description of an expanding genetic and clinical syndrome. Muscle Nerve. 2004; 29: 323–328.

Lilleker JB, Keh YS, Roncaroli F, et al. Metabolic myopathies. Pract Neurol. 2018; 18(1): 14–26.

McConchie SM, Coakley J, Edwards RH, et al. Molecular heterogeneity in McArdle's disease. Biochim Biophys. 1990; Acta. 1096: 26–32.

Mellies U, Lofaso F. Pompe disease: a neuromuscular disease with respiratory muscle involvement. Resp Med. 2009; 103: 477–484.

Sharma MC, Schultze C, von Moers A, et al. Delayed or late-onset type II glycogenosis with globular inclusions. Acta Neuropathol. 2005; 110: 151–157.

Usuki F, Takenaga S, Higuchi I, et al. Morphologic findings in biopsied skeletal muscle and cultured fibroblasts from a female patient with Danon's disease (lysosomal glycogen storage disease without acid maltase deficiency). J Neurol Sci. 1994; 127: 54–60.

Woo M, Chung SJ, Nonaka I. Perifascicular atrophic fibers in childhood dermatomyositis with particular reference to mitochondrial changes. J Neurol Sci. 1988; 88: 133–143.

CHAPTER 20

INFLAMMATORY MYOPATHY

Contents

Inflammatory myopathy (IM) comprises a diverse group of acquired skeletal muscle diseases often occurring in complex clinical settings. It is a diagnostic challenge in clinical practice that usually requires multidisciplinary expertise to reach an accurate diagnosis. Since the 1990s, the classification of IMs has been limited by specific pathological variants, defined by Bohan and Peter et al. These variants include polymyositis (PM), dermatomyositis (DM), and inclusion body myositis (IBM). The only distinction between these conditions is the skin involvement. Several attempts have been made to enroll serological autoantibodies in the diagnostic workup. Love et al. and Troyanove et al., at the end of the nineteenth century, created a novel classification of IMs based on autoantibody profiles. Unfortunately, it has recently been proven that fewer than 50% of patients with IMs present with known antibodies, and that classification lacks the association with morphological data. In 2003, immune-mediated myopathy (IMM) was included in the classification of IMs as a new entity.

The Pestronk criteria were the best-integrated classification system in the context of IM diagnosis. He translated pathological findings into well-recognizable terms that combined the morphological data with clinical and laboratory results. This traditional method of diagnosis is still valid despite the novel publications for myositis classification that have been formally accepted by the European League Against Rheumatism/American College of Rheumatology. The diagnostic criteria are collected to lead to a "definite," "probable," or "possible" diagnosis. Although these criteria revealed high sensitivity and specificity measures, they still lack the sufficient data required for a reliable diagnosis.

To date, there is no widely accepted consensus regarding the classification of IMs. Allenbach et al. (2017), Satoh et al. (2017), Carstens and Schmidt et al. (2018), and Landberg et al (2016) have reviewed the IM classification system and made profuse modifications to its morphological and diagnostic aspects. Allenbach et al. integrated the autoantibodies into the clinical and pathological variants of myositis. This recent integration was to date the most successful classification system for myositis. Carstens and Schmidt et al. have revisited the classification and updated the actual components of myositis variants. They also concluded that polymyositis (PM), is a non-existing disease that now falls into the category of overlap myositis or on the polymyositis/dermatomyositis (PM/DM) spectrum.

The majority of IMs have an autoimmune background, thus the precise mechanism of the immune response in their groups has not been fully characterized. However, we can conclude that all IMs are almost idiopathic. Cellular immune mechanisms include cytotoxic CD8+ T-cells that make cell-to-cell contact with muscle fibers and exert their cytotoxic granules with granzyme B in the direction of muscle fibers. Mediators of the innate immune system have also been noted in myositis, and the expression of toll-like receptors is present on muscle fiber sarcolemma. Non-immune stress mechanisms were also discovered in myositis pathogenesis in which ER stress, NFκB-activation, and free radicals were associated. Moreover, the HLA 8.1 haplotype has been identified as a risk factor for myositis in a genome-wide analysis.

In IBM, autophagic activity in the form of amyloid aggregation recently has been found to be associated with some genetic variants of VCP, SQSTM1, and FYCO1 mutations.

Secondary inflammatory myopathies are very rare and associated with particular etiologies such as chronic infections, malignancy, and chronic systemic diseases.

IMs can affect any age, but some entities are more likely to affect adult more than children. Most cases clinically present with pain and weakness of different muscle distributions, more often the proximal muscles of the lower limbs rather than upper limbs. Typical complaints include problems in walking and climbing stairs or lifting an object above the head. Other organs such as skin and the lungs are frequently involved, supporting that IMs are systemic inflammatory diseases. CK level is always elevated (10–50 fold) beyond the normal range because of the necrotizing nature of IMs. Electromyography (EMG) may show irritative myopathic patterns in the form of fibrillations, contractions, and positive sharp waves; however, EMG may sometimes show non-specific results. At this stage, the clinician needs a muscle biopsy to confirm the diagnosis.

The obstacle with muscle biopsy is that it is not only used as a confirmatory test, but it is sometimes difficult to discern what type of myositis is seen in the biopsy. Overlapping clinical phenotypes and autoantibodies among IMs entities make the diagnosis difficult to establish. Indeed, the clinician must combine all findings together to reach a final conclusion.

Numerous studies have analyzed the relevance of autoantibody phenotypes with clinical presentation and outcome. These antibodies have subcellular targets that are often directed against proteins associated with RNA transcription. They could be either specific to some types of myositis (myositis-specific antibodies, MSA) or associated with different variants (myositis-associated antibodies, MAA). This is considered a diagnostic challenge as the MAAs can be detected in several types of myositis with different combinations, which makes the diagnosis more sophisticated. Classifying IMs by autoantibodies may be confusing as many myositis overlap. In conclusion, the arbitrary distinction between MSA and MAA appears to be rather obsolete.

In muscle biopsy, myositis is histologically characterized by the presence of myonecrosis, regeneration, and inflammation (**Figure 20.1a**). It is sometimes difficult to reach a specific diagnosis by only hematoxylin and eosin (H&E) stain and the pathologist may sign the case as either inflammatory myositis (non-specific) or necrotizing myopathy. Sub-diagnosis comments, where pathologists can explain the histopathological findings within the clinical context, are important for the clinician.

The definitive features of myositis are different from disease to disease. Necrotic fibers in PM are subtle and may be the only features seen, which may mimic other types of IMNM or muscular dystrophies. In dermatomyositis (DM), perifascicular pathology (including atrophy, necrosis, or regeneration) is considered a pathognomonic sign in all DM variants particularly the juvenile types (**Figure 20.1b**). Perifascicular pathology may also occur in non-DM diseases such as IM with perimysial pathology (IMPP) or anti-RNA synthetase myositis spectrum (ARS).

Rimmed vacuoles, protein aggregates, and mitochondrial abnormalities are restricted to IBM (**Figure 20.2**). However, perifascicular COX-negative fiber is commonly observed in cases of DM. This occurs due to mitochondrial dysfunction in the perifascicular degenerated fibers.

Scattered studies reported rimmed vacuoles in DM, and for unknown mechanism.

The inflammation in myositis is variable. It can be histiocytic (CD68+ macrophages), T-cell lymphocytic (CD4+ or CD8+ cells), or rarely B-cell infiltration. Its distribution also varies in each myositis. For example, IBM has more predominant CD8+ cytotoxic cells compared to DM and PM. IMNM would have more CD68+ macrophages in the perimysium than CD4+ T-cells.

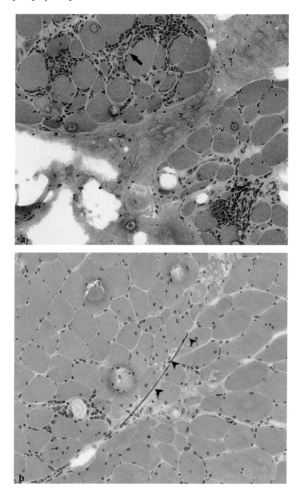

Figure 20.1 H&E sections from patients with inflammatory myopathies. **(a)** A section from a 33-year-old man with inflammatory myositis shows severe endomysial inflammation (*black arrow*). **(b)** A section from a 27-year-old woman with anti-M2 dermatomyositis reveals a perifascicular atrophy and necrosis (*arrowheads*). ×25.

In immune myopathy with abundant macrophages (IMAM), the predominant inflammatory cells are CD68+ macrophages diffusely present in the perimysium. The site of inflammation in muscle tissue could be endomysial, perimysial, and/or perivascular. This can help to differentiate between some IM variants. PM, IBM, and some patterns of OMs may show inflammatory cells invading non-necrotic fibers (**Figure 20.2f**).

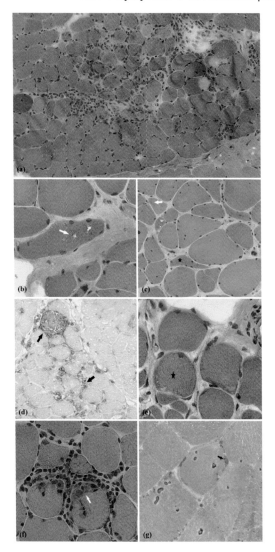

Figure 20.2 Sections from a 50-year-old male patient show histological features of inclusion body myositis. **(a)** H&E section shows marked inflammatory necrotizing myopathy with endomysial and perimysial inflammation and fibrosis. **(b)** Rimmed vacuole (*white arrow*). **(c)** Section shows cytoplasmic body (*white arrow*) and small angulated fiber due to neuropathic involvement (***). **(d)** Section shows predominant endomysial CD8+ T-cell inflammation (*black arrows*). **(e)** Muscle fiber with mitochondrial abnormality (***). **(f)** Inflammatory cells invading non-necrotic fibers (*white arrow*). **(g)** Toluidine-epoxy thick section shows tiny inclusions in the muscle fiber nuclei (*black arrow*). Different magnifications (×15–×40).

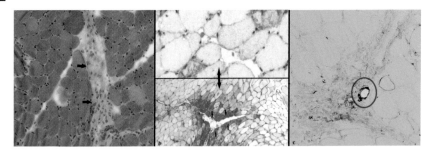

Figure 20.3 Histological sections from different patients with inflammatory myopathies. **(a)** H&E section from a 43-year-old man with IMPM shows perimysial fragmentation (*black arrows*). **(b)** MHC class-I sections from a female patient with dermatomyositis show either scattered sarcolemmal expression of muscle fibers or perifascicular expression (*black arrowheads*). *Reprinted with permission from Dr. Robert Hammond, Western University, Canada.* **(c)** Same patient as part **(b)**, shows MAC-C5b-9 deposition mainly in microvessels.

Perimysial fragmentation, a histological sign observed in some types of myositis, is characterized by degenerating muscle fibers in perimysium with predominant macrophage infiltration (**Figure 20.3a**). It can be associated with anti-*Mi2*-DM, anti-*SRP*, IMPP, and statin-induced myopathies.

The most significant application of immunohistochemistry (IHC) in IMs is the assessment of MHC class-I expression in muscle fibers. In normal muscle, MHC class-I is expressed in normal capillaries, which can be used as a tissue control. In abnormal muscle, MHC class-I is detected in the sarcolemma of myositis cases. However, sarcolemmal MHC class-I expression is not specific for IMs and has been detected in other non-inflammatory myopathies such as LGMD-2B and GSD-II.

The use of MHC class-I in IMs can help pathologists to determine the specific type of myositis (**Table 20.1**). Perifascicular MHC-I expression is common in all variants of DM but also has been noted in cases of anti-synthetase myositis such as the anti-Jo-1 and anti-PL-7 PM/DM spectrum (**Figure 20.3b**). Widespread expression of MHC class-I in muscle fibers is commonly seen in IBM and non-DM variants.

Membrane attack complex (MAC; C5b-9) is commonly used as another parameter to assess cases with myositis. MAC is expressed in endomysial microvessels of DM (**Figure 20.3c**). MAC has also been detected in scattered necrotic fibers of DM and other variants.

Among all types of IMs, myositis with anti-TIFI-γ, anti-NXP2, and anti-HMGCoR antibodies is associated with malignancy, most commonly lung cancers and lymphoma. Certainly, all patients with newly diagnosed myositis should go for a CT scan or MRI of the chest and abdomen. Tumor

Table 20.1 Integrated classification of inflammatory myopathies (IM).

IM subtype	Autoantibodies	Inflammation site	Inflammation type	Perifascicular pathology	MHC expression pattern	MAC-C5b9 pattern	Fibrosis fragmentation	Pathognomonic signs	Associated diseases
Inflammatory myositis syndromes									
Polymyositis (no longer exists)	Anti tRNA synthetase								
	Anti-Jo1/PL-7	PM/EM	CD4 > CD8	Rare	Perifascicular+/-	Perimysium	EMF	None	ILD
	Non-anti tRNA synthetase								
	PM-Scl/Ku/SRP	EM + INNF	CD8 > CD4	No	Widespread	None	EMF	Severe NM	Scleroderma/ILD
Polymyositis dermatomyositis spectrum	Anti tRNA synthetase								
	Anti-Jo1/PL-7	PM/EM	CD4 > CD8	Yes	Perifascicular+/-	Perimysium	EMF	None	ILD/GIT upset
	Non-anti tRNA synthetase								
	MDA5	PM	CD4 > CD68	No	Widespread	None	PMF	None	ILD/MH
Dermatomyositis									
Classical adult	Mi-2	PV/PM	CD4 > CD8	Yes	Perifascicular	Capillaries	PMF/PMFr	TRI/MxA+	Rash
Juvenile	TIFI-γ Juvenile	PV/PM/EM	CD20 > CD4	Yes	Perifascicular+/-	Capillaries	PMF	TRI/PME	Rash/cancers
	SAE	PM/EM	CD4 > CD8	Rare	Widespread	None	PMF	None	Rash/ILD
	NXP2 Juvenile	PM/EM	CD4 > CD8	Yes	Perifascicular	Capillaries	PMF	None	Calcinosis
Amyopathic DM	MDA5	PM	CD4 > CD68	No	Widespread	None	PMF	None	Rash/ILD/MH
	TIFI-γ/SAE	PM/EM	CD4 > CD8	Yes	Perifascicular	Capillaries	PMF	TRI	Rash/cancers
IMAM	TNFRSF1 gene	PM	CD68 > CD20	No	Widespread	Capillaries	PMF	TRI	Rash/arthritis
Inclusion body myositis (IBM)	5NT1A 5NTC1A Ro52	EM/PV/PM INNF	CD8 > CD4 CD68+	No	Widespread Scattered	None	EMF	RV/ RRF +/- Cox (-) fibers TFI	SLE/SD/CLL polyneuropathy
Immune medicated necrotizing myopathies (IMNM)									
IMPP	Anti-Jo1	PM	CD4 > CD68	Rare	Perifascicular+/-	Perimysium	PMF/PMFr	INFI/PSC	ILD/RD/MH
INM-SRP	SRP	PM	Rare	No	Perifascicular+/-	Sarcocapillary	PMF/PMFr	PSC	CM/dysphagia
RIIM	NXP2	PM	Rare	No	Widespread	Capillaries	PMF	Necrotic BV	Rash/cancers
Statin myopathy	HMG-CoR	PM	CD68 > CD4	No	MHC+ NNF	None	PMF/PMFr	None	Cancers
Non-specific type of primary myositis									
BCIM	Anti-AcH	PV/PM	CD20 > CD4	No	Widespread	Endomysium	PMF	MxA+	MGD/RA

Abbreviations: OM: overlap myositis. MHC: major histocompatibility. MAC: membrane attack complex. ILD: interstitial lung disease. NM: necrotizing myopathy. ARS: anti-aminoacyl tRNA-synthetase antibody. Mi-2: helicase protein part of NuRD complex. MDA5: melanoma differentiation-associated gene 5. SRP: signal recognition particle antibody. TRI: tubuloreticular inclusion. PM: perimysium. EM: endomysium. PV: perivascular. PMF: perimysial fibrosis. EMF: endomysial fibrosis. PMFr: perimysial fragmentation. PME: perimysial edema. MxA: myxovirus resistance A. INNF: invading non-necrotic fibers. IMAM: inflammatory myopathy with abundant macrophage. TIFI: transcription intermediary factor 1-gamma. NXP2: nuclear matrix protein 2. SAE: small ubiquitin-like modifier activating enzyme. SD: Sjogren disease. NNF: non-necrotic fibers. INFI: intranuclear filamentous inclusion. CM: cardiomyopathy. PSC: pipestem capillaries. RD: Raynaud's disease. MH: mechanical hand. RV: rimmed vacuoles. RRF: ragged red fiber. TFI: tubulofilamentous inclusion. SLE: systemic lupus erythematosus. CLL: chronic lymphocytic leukemia. Sarcocapillary: sarcocplasmic and capillaries. IMPP: immune myopathy with perimysial pathology. RIIM: regional ischemic immune myopathy. BV: blood vessels. BCIM: brachiocervical inflammatory myopathy. MGD: myasthenia gravis disease. RA: rheumatoid arthritis. HMGCoR: hydroxy-3-methylglutaryl-coenzyme A reductase.

screening should also be repeated every year for at least 3 years, after confirming the diagnosis.

Although several papers have explained the histopathological features of IM variants in association with autoantibodies, the need to have fixed classification guidelines is paramount. This consensus would assist the clinician in patient treatment plans and prognosis. We propose here a comprehensive classification of IMs that incorporates clinical information, morphological features, antibody profiles, and molecular data, as well as the previous classification systems in the literature. This assemblage focuses on recent advances in myositis that can be used as guidelines to diagnose patients with inflammatory myopathy. **Figure 20.4** and **Figure 20.5** summarize this comprehensive and integrated classification of IMs with an illustrated approach to diagnose cases with myositis via muscle biopsy. **Figure 20.9** illustrates a structural diagram of all types of myositis with their associated autoantibodies and characteristic features of each disease.

IMs are classified, based on our system, into primary and secondary type. The primary IM is collectively named *inflammatory myositis* or *idiopathic inflammatory myopathies* (IIMs). It includes PM, DM, PM/DM spectrum, IBM, and immune-mediated myopathies (IMMs). PM/DM spectrum and IMMs are parts of ARS spectrum, including anti-Jo1, anti-PL7, and anti-PL12. Dermatomyositis (DM) is categorized into classical adult-onset DM and juvenile type DM. IMM is subcategorized into different controversial variants including immune myopathy with perimysial pathology (IMPP), anti-HMGCoR myopathy (statin-myopathy), anti-SRP (single recognition particle) myopathy, and regional ischemic immune myopathy (RIIM). IMPP is a controversial entity recently replaced by anti-Jo1 myopathy.

Other rare entities under IMs, not included in the above-mentioned classification, are immune myopathy with abundant macrophages (IMAM) and brachiocervical myopathies (BCM).

All IM groups are summarized in **Table 20.1**. This table distinguishes all variants based on characteristic associated autoantibodies, inflammation site and types, perifascicular pathology, MHC/MAC expression, and associated clinical conditions. The diagnosis will be very conclusive if the pathological approach illustrated in **Figure 20.5** is followed.

Secondary IM is a rare group of muscle diseases that is subclassified into granulomatous and non-granulomatous inflammation; the latter occurs due to chronic infection, malignancy, or is associated with some chronic diseases.

Myopathic features with focal inflammation, not part of primary IMs, include different types of muscular dystrophies such as LGMD-2B, FHMD,

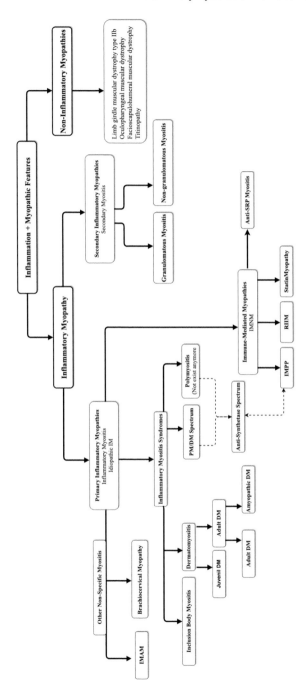

Figure 20.4 General classification of inflammatory myopathies. PM: polymyositis. DM: dermatomyositis. IMPP: immune myopathy with perimysial pathology. SRP: signal recognition particle antibody. RIIM: regional ischemic immune myopathy. IMAM: inflammatory myopathy with abundant macrophage.

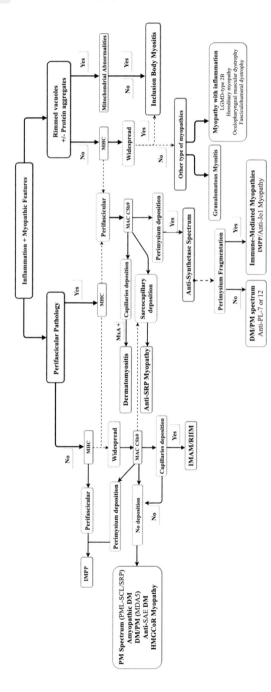

Figure 20.5 Pathological approach to diagnose inflammatory myositis. LGMD: limb-girdle muscular dystrophy. MHC: major histocompatibility. MAC: membrane attack complex. PM: polymyositis. DM: dermatomyositis. IMPP: immune myopathy with perimysial pathology. MxA: myxovirus resistance A. MDA5: melanoma differentiation-associated gene 5. SAE: small ubiquitin-like modifier activating enzyme. SRP: signal recognition particle antibody. IMAM: inflammatory myopathy with abundant macrophage. Sarcocapillary: sarcoplasmic and capillaries. RIIM: regional ischemic immune myopathy. HMGCoR: hydroxy-3-methylglutaryl-coenzyme A reductase.

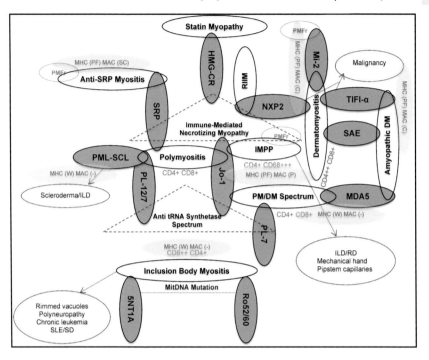

Figure 20.9 Structural diagram of IM variants, which illustrates myositis syndromes with their associated autoantibodies and distinct pathological features of each disease. DM: dermatomyositis. PM: polymyositis. P: perimysium. PF: perifascicular. W: widespread. PMFr: perimysial fragmentation. SC: sarcocapillary. MHC: major histocompatibility. MAC: membrane attack complex. Mi-2: helicase protein part of NuRD complex. MDA5: melanoma differentiation-associated gene 5. SRP: signal recognition particle antibody. TIFI: transcription intermediary factor 1-gamma. NXP2: nuclear matrix protein 2. SAE: small ubiquitin-like modifier activating enzyme. ILD: interstitial lung disease. SD: Sjogren disease. RD: Raynaud's disease. SLE: systemic lupus erythematosus. RIIM: regional ischemic immune myopathy.

and OPMD. This should be excluded by histopathology and immunostain labelling.

For a reliable diagnosis of myositis, the institution receiving the muscle biopsy should have a capable neuromuscular team that can provide robust clinical information of patient history and be able to perform a broad autoantibody assay. **Figure 20.5** illustrates an integrated approach to diagnose cases with IMs.

20.1 Polymyositis (PM, Adermatopathic Myositis)

The diagnosis of polymyositis (PM) is probably obsolete, because it may encompass many different diseases. It is the rarest form of myositis, and some authors even question its existence. It is generally accepted that none of the reported antibodies of PM were actually associated with the disease spectrum. PM as a separate entity is undoubtedly non-existent and should be considered only if other well-defined diseases have been excluded. However, the disease should be re-classified as overlap myositis or adermatopathic myositis. Patients present clinically with a subacute proximal rather symmetric myopathy without skin symptoms, no family history of muscle disease, and after having ruled out toxic, viral, and muscular dystrophy conditions. The usual feature of the diseases is necrotizing myopathy with very minimal endomysial T-cell inflammation invading non-necrotic muscle fibers (**Figure 20.6**). There is a widespread expression of MHC class-I in the entire fiber. No cytological vacuolations, mitochondrial aggregation, or perifascicular pathology have

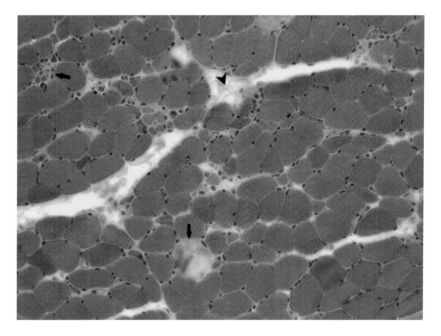

Figure 20.6 H&E section from a 34-year-old man with inflammatory myositis and anti-SRP antibody. There is evidence of necrotizing myopathy without inflammation (*black arrows*). There is also a focal area of perimysial fragmentation (*black arrowhead*). ×25.

been reported. The majority of reported cases in the literature support that anti-SRP and anti-PML-SCL autoantibodies are closely related to PM and associated with treatment-resistant forms.

20.2 Dermatomyositis (DM)

Dermatomyositis (DM) is characterized by dermatomyopathic change and inflammation. The patient clinically presents with muscle symptoms with or without dermatological features (Gottron papules and heliotrope rash). The classical features of DM in muscle biopsy are the presence of myonecrosis, regeneration, perimysial or perivascular inflammation, and with or without perifascicular pathology; the latter is well-visualized by perifascicular COX (–) staining or perifascicular MHC class-I expression (**Figure 20.3b**). MAC is strongly deposited in the capillaries with rare sarcolemmal staining (**Figure 20.3c**). Rimmed vacuoles have been identified in few cases with dermatomyositis. The mechanism is not yet understood. However, some of these cases presented with IBM features.

The inflammation in DM is always CD4+ T-cells rather than CD8+ cytotoxic T-cells. CD68 macrophages are variable. Many reports demonstrated that immunohistochemical staining for MxA (myxovirus resistance A) protein is a sensitive marker for DM more than the perifascicular pathology and MAC deposition. The most pathognomonic sign of DM is the presence of tubuloreticular inclusions (TRI) in endothelial cells, seen ultrastructurally (**Figure 12.1b; Chapter 12**).

Several autoantibodies have been reported in the DM spectrum. The most common and longest known autoantibody associated with the classical form is anti-Mi-2 antibody, which is found in up to 20% of patients with DM (**Table 20.1**). This variant presents with classic skin rash, perifascicular pathology, and MAC deposition in capillaries, as well as good response to steroid, and good prognosis. Juvenile type DM is associated with anti-NXP2 antibody (nuclear matrix protein 2) and anti-TIFI-γ (transcription intermediary factor 1-gamma). Children usually present with myopathy, skin features, and swallowing difficulties. In adults, 30%–40% of cases having anti-TIFI-γ and anti-NXP2 are associated with malignancy,

Anti-MDA5 antibody (melanoma differentiation-associated protein 5) was first identified as CADM-140 antigen. It is a cytoplasmic RNA-specific helicase that belongs to a family of retinoic acid-inducible gene (RIG) I-like receptors. It is associated with amyopathic DM or DM/PM spectrum (non-ARS). These patients are clinically asymptomatic with minimal skin features. There is no perifascicular pathology, but MHC class-I may show either widespread or perifascicular expression. The majority of these cases have high prevalence of rapid progressive interstitial lung disease leading to early death.

20.3 Immune-Mediated Necrotizing Myopathy (IMNM)

IMNM is a rare entity recently involved in the classification of IMs. It is characterized clinically with rapid disease course. The CK level is usually very high with 20–50 folds. Three autoantibodies have been shown to be associated with IMNM: anti-SRP, anti-HMGCoR, and anti-Jo1 antibodies. Anti-SRP has been explained before as a variant of PM that presents with severe necrotizing myopathy with absent or very minimal significant inflammation. It may be associated clinically with dysphagia, cardiomyopathy, and interstitial lung disease.

Anti-HMGCoR is another variant commonly associated with statin-induced myopathy or some rare malignancies. This is explained in detail in *Chapter 18*.

Immune myopathy with perimysial pathology (IMPP) has recently been categorized as anti-tRNA synthetase syndrome because of its association with anti-Jo1 antibody. The disease course is progressive and aggressive and associated with remarkable changes in muscle biopsy. The predominate histological features of IMPP are perimysial CD68+ inflammation, fibrosis, and perimysial fragmentation (**Figure 20.3a**). Perifascicular MHC class-I expression can be detected in muscle fibers, sarcolemma, and capillaries. MAC complement is restricted to sarcolemma. IMPP has no specific ultrastructural features. Pipestem capillaries or intranuclear filamentous inclusions might be seen. Pipestem capillaries are characterized by thickened microangiopathy where it shows PAS deposition in the internal layer. It can also be associated with other chronic diseases such as diabetes.

20.4 Overlap Myositis (OM)

Overlap myositis is a controversial spectrum of IMs that share two or more variants of myositis (PM, PM/DM, and IMNM). The most common overlapping condition is anti-synthetase syndrome (AS), a distinct special variant of myositis-associated autoantibodies. It consists of a typical collection of clinical symptoms including myositis, Raynaud's disease (RD), arthritis, mechanic's hands (MH), interstitial lung disease (ILD), and presence of anti-tRNA synthetase autoantibodies. The most common of the eight anti-synthetase antibodies is anti-Jo1 antibody. Anti-PL-7 and anti-PL-12 are other rare variants found in PM or the PM/DM spectrum (**Table 20.1**).

Anti-Jo1 antibody syndrome was previously categorized as IMPP, but recent advances in myositis classification have updated this theory. Although IMPP is no longer present and all have been re-classified as anti-synthetase syndrome, some diagnosticians still use this controversial term. The histopathological features of IMPP or anti-synthetase syndrome have been explained above and also summarized in **Table 20.1**. Other types of antibodies such as anti-SSA/Ro52/Ro60 and anti-SS-B/La, are present in Sjogren's disease (SD), systemic lupus erythematosus (SLE), and systemic sclerosis (SS). Anti-Ro52 is often present in conjunction with anti-synthetase antibodies. These double-positive patients have a higher risk of malignancy and a poorer prognosis.

In summary, OM is the largest subgroup of IMs that always present with two or more autoantibodies or myositis variants. These cases are difficult to diagnose and need careful clinical, pathological, and laboratory correlations.

20.5 Inclusion Body Myositis (IBM)

The clinical presentation of inclusion body myositis (INM) is distinct from all other forms of myositis. The weakness is always slowly progressive, asymmetrical, and affecting distal more than proximal muscles. The typical pattern of muscle involvement includes weakness of the long finger flexors, quadriceps muscle, tibialis anterior, and, rarely, spreads to involve other muscles of the arms and legs. The disease commonly presents with swallowing difficulties. The age-onset is variable, but the disease affects adults ages 50 years and older, in particular men more than women. Skin involvement has never been reported in IBM.

IBM can be associated with some chronic conditions such SLE, SD, CLL, and polyneuropathy. The most common antibody associated with IBM is cN1A (5NT1A/5NTC1A), which is 95% sensitive. Patients presenting with these antibodies may have progressive disease and a high mortality rate. The histological picture encompasses myopathic features in the form of myonecrosis, regeneration, and scattered hypertrophic fibers. There is an invasion of non-necrotic muscle fibers by endomysial cytotoxic CD8+ T-cells (**Figure 20.2d–f**). The MHC class-I is expressed in the sarcolemma and always widespread. MAC deposition is absent. The pathognomonic sign of IBM in muscle biopsy is the presence of rimmed vacuoles and cytoplasmic protein aggregates such as cytoplasmic bodies (**Figure 20.2b–c**). Congophilic inclusions are more easily detected by Congo red staining viewed under rhodamine optics rather than polarized light. The vacuoles can also be highlighted with P62, Tau, and TDP-43 stains. IBM can also present as neuromyopathic changes due to the polyneuropathic component of the disease.

Ultrastructurally, tubulofilamentous inclusions (TFI) in myonuclei might be seen. Signs of mitochondrial dysfunction due to MitDNA mutations have been observed in several cases of IBM. These features are histologically described as ragged-red fibers and COX-negative fibers (**Figure 20.2e**), and abnormal mitochondrial paracrystallin inclusions in EM sections (**Figure 12.1i, Chapter 12**).

20.6 Granulomatous Myositis

Granulomatous myositis is a very rare inflammatory condition characterized histologically by granulomatous or granulomatoid inflammation. It is usually seen as a manifestation of sarcoidosis, but isolated granulomatous myositis may occur. Some cases of IBM have been misdiagnosed as granulomatous myositis. Granulomatous myositis can also be associated with graft-versus-host disease, chronic infection (tuberculosis or brucellosis) and rarely lymphoma. T-cell leukemia may mimic granulomatous inflammation in muscle biopsy. The patient always presents with chronic muscle weakness and moderate elevation of CK level. The hallmark histological feature in muscle biopsy is granuloma with multinucleated giant cells or Langhans cells.

20.7 Treated Myositis in Muscle Biopsy

Many clinicians send muscle biopsies after starting patients on steroid therapy. Unfortunately, this leads to inaccurate results, because the steroid therapy may mask the inflammation and mimic other types of myopathic diseases. Although there is no exact estimated time of inflammation healing after starting the therapy, many expert pathologists expect that the inflammation may not appear if the biopsy is taken 3 days after steroid therapy. It is very important that muscle biopsy being taken before starting the patient treatment. In such cases, MHC class-I and MAC expression can be used to rule out IMs. MHC class-I sarcoplasmic expression with or without MAC deposition in capillaries shifts the diagnosis toward IMs. Predominant type-II atrophy is commonly seen in patients receiving steroid therapy.

CLINICAL CASE #1

A 16-year-old healthy female patient presented to the neuromuscular clinic with acute onset of generalized body weakness for 1 week. She denies any dysphagia, skin rash, or respiratory symptoms. Physical examination is unremarkable except for reduced muscle strength in upper limbs more than lower limbs. The reflexes are intact. Serum CK level is 1160 IU/L. Liver enzymes are within normal range. EMG/NCT show irritative myopathic patterns. There is no evidence of neurogenic patterns in NCT.

Based on the Above Findings, What is Your Differential Diagnosis?

A biopsy is done from her right biceps muscle. Histological sections are illustrated in **Figure 20.7**.

- Explain the histopathological findings.
- What is your likely diagnosis?

Interpretation

H&E section shows marked myopathic features with necrosis, regeneration, and evidence of severe inflammation (**Figure 20.7**). The inflammation looks granulomatoid with perimysial, endomysial, and perivascular distributions. No definitive perifascicular pathology is identified. There is no neuropathic change, cytological vacuolations, or mitochondrial abnormalities. There is no perimysial fragmentation. The inflammation is predominantly highlighted with CD4 and CD68 markers but not with CD8 (**Figure 20.7**). MHC class-I is expressed in some sarcocapillaries. Ultrastructural examination of the muscle tissue shows unremarkable findings.

Because granulomatoid inflammation mimics granuloma, screening for chronic infections such as tuberculosis or brucellosis is ruled out clinicopathologically. The patient has no sarcoid manifestations.

In summary, the histopathological features are consistent with idiopathic inflammatory myositis. The specific variant is difficult to establish here. Therefore, an autoantibodies profile is clinically recommended. Current differential variants include juvenile DM (anti-NXP2 or anti-TIFI-γ) or overlap myositis.

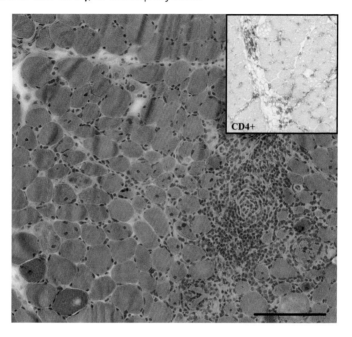

Figure 20.7 Histological sections from a 16-year-old girl with severe granulomatoid and lymphocytic inflammation. CD4+ T-cells are the predominant inflammatory cell type. ×20.

CLINICAL CASE #2

A 38-year-old woman presented to the rheumatology clinic with 6 months history of fatigue, dysphagia, and slowly progressive proximal weakness of upper and lower limbs. There is no skin rash. Physical examination reveals reduced muscle power in the upper and lower limbs, proximal more than distal, and without muscle wasting. The reflexes are intact. Her body examination only shows a physical sign of mechanical hands. Chest X-ray reveals minimal infiltrates in the right and left lungs, of undetermined significance. EMG/NCT reveal evidence of irritable myopathy.

Based on the Above Findings, What is Your Differential Diagnosis?

A biopsy is done from her left deltoid muscle. Histological sections are illustrated in **Figure 20.8.**

- Explain the histopathological findings.
- What is your likely diagnosis?

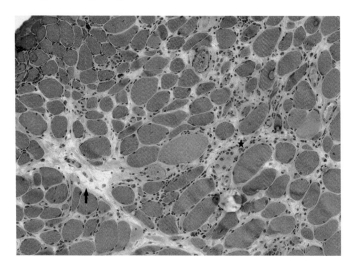

Figure 20.8 H&E section from a 38-year-old woman with immune-mediated necrotizing myopathy. There is marked perimysial and endomysial fibrosis (*), and perimysial fragmentation (*black arrow*). ×25.

Interpretation

H&E section shows marked variation in muscle size and shape. There is evidence of myopathic features in the form of necrosis and regeneration. Minimal histiocytic inflammation in the perimysium is noted. There is severe perimysial and endomysial fibrosis and perimysial fragmentation is clearly visible (**Figure 20.8**).

This histopathological description is consistent with the diagnosis of immune-mediated necrotizing myopathy, likely IMPP.

An antibody profile screen is performed and revealed anti-Jo1 autoantibody in high titration. This result is associated with anti-Jo1 synthetase myositis, a part of IMNM spectrum.

References

Allenbach Y, Benveniste O, Goebel HH, Stenzel W. Integrated classification of inflammatory myopathies. Neuropathol App Neurobiol. 2017; 43(1): 62–81.

Allenbach Y, Leroux G, Suarez-Calvet X, Preusse C, Gallardo E, Hervier B, et al. Dermatomyositis with or without anti-melanoma differentiation-associated gene 5 antibodies: common interferon signature but distinct NOS2 expression. Am J Pathol. 2016; 186: 691–700.

Alshehri A, Choksi R, Bucelli R, Pestronk A. Myopathy with anti-HMGCR antibodies: perimysium and myofiber pathology. Neurol Neuroimmunol Neuroinflamm. 2015; 2: e124.

Bucelli RC, Pestronk A. Immune myopathies with perimysial pathology: clinical and laboratory features. Neurol Neuroimmunol Neuroinflamm. 2018; 5(2): e434.

Cai C, Alshehri A, Choksi R, Pestronk A. Regional ischemic immune myopathy: a paraneoplastic dermatomyopathy. J Neuropathol Exp Neurol. 2014; 73(12): 1126–1133.

Carstens PO, Schmidt J. Diagnosis, pathogenesis and treatment of myositis: recent advances. Clin Exp Immunol. 2014; 175(3): 349–358.

Chahin N, Engel AG. Correlation of muscle biopsy, clinical course, and outcome in PM and sporadic IBM. Neurology. 2008; 70(6): 418–424.

Christopher-Stine L, Casciola-Rosen LA, Hong G, Chung T, Corse AM, Mammen AL. A novel autoantibody recognizing 200-kd and 100-kd proteins is associated with an immune-mediated necrotizing myopathy. Arthritis Rheum. 2010; 62(9): 2757–2766.

Dalakas MC. Inflammatory muscle diseases. N Engl J Med. 2015; 372(18): 1734–1747.

Dalakas MC. Polymyositis, dermatomyositis and inclusion body myositis. N Engl J Med. 1991; 325: 1487–1498.

Das L, Blumberg PC, Manavis J, Limaye VS. Major histocompatibility complex class I and II expression in idiopathic inflammatory myopathy. Appl Immunohistochem Mol Morphol. 2013; 21(6): 539–542.

Garel B, Barete S, Rigolet A, Le Pelletier F, Benveniste O, Hervier B. Severe adult dermatomyositis with unusual calcinosis. Rheumatology (Oxford). 2015; 54: 2024.

Goebels N, Michaelis D, Engelhardt M, Huber S, Bender A, Pongratz D, et al. Differential expression of perforin in muscle-infiltrating T cells in polymyositis and dermatomyositis. J Clin Invest. 1996; 97(12): 2905–2910.

Gonzales PS, Grau JM. Diagnosis and classification of granulomatous myositis. Autoimmun Rev. 2014; 13(4–5): 372–374.

Graca CR, Kouyoimdjian JA. MHC class I antigens, CD4 and CD8 expressions in polymyositis and dermatomyositis. Rev Bras Reumatol. 2015; 55(3): 203–208.

Gunawardena H, Wedderburn LR, Chinoy H, Betteridge ZE, North J, Ollier WE, et al. Autoantibodies to a 140-kd protein in juvenile dermatomyositis are associated with calcinosis. Arthritis Rheum. 2009; 60(6): 1807–1814.

Gunawardena H. The clinical features of myositis-associated autoantibodies: a review. Clin Rev Allergy Immunol. 2017; 52(1): 45–57.

Guttsches AK, Brady S, Krause K, Maerkens A, Uszkoreit J, Eisenacher M, et al. Proteomics of rimmed vacuoles define new risk allele in inclusion body myositis. Ann Neurol. 2017; 81(2): 227–239.

Hirkakta M, Suwa A, Nagai S, et al. Anti-KS: Identification of autoantibodies to asparaginyl-transfer RNSA synthetase associated with interstitial lung disease. J Immunol. 1999; 162: 2315–2320.

Hussenbux A, Hofer M, Steuer A. Statin-induced necrotizing autoimmune myopathy: importance of early recognition. Br J Hosp Med (Lonf). 2017: 78(6): 352–353.

Ichimura Y, Matsushita T, Hamaguchi Y, Kaji K, et al. Anti-NXP2 autoantibodies in adult patients with idiopathic inflammatory myopathies: possible association with malignancy. Ann Rheum Dis. 2012; 71: 710–713.

Kao AH, Lacomis D, Lucas M, Fertig N, Oddis CV. Anti-signal recognition particle autoantibody in patients with and patients without idiopathic inflammatory myopathy. Arthritis Rheum. 2004; 50: 209–215.

Levian M, Goyal N, Mozaffar T. Sporadic inclusion body myositis misdiagnosed as idiopathic granulomatous myositis. Neuromuscul Disord. 2016; 26(11): 741–843.

Lilleker JB, Rietveld A, Pye SR, Mariampillai K, Benveniste O, Peeters MT, et al. Cytosolic 5'-nucleotidase 1A autoantibody profile and clinical characteristics in inclusion body myositis. Ann Rheum Dis. 2017; 76(5): 862–868.

Limaya VS, Blumbergs P. The prevalence of rimmed vacuoles in biopsy-proven dermatomyositis. Muscle Nerve. 2010; 41(2): 288–289.

Love LA, Leff RL, Fraser DD, Targoff IN, Dalakas M, Plotz PH, Miller FW. A new approach to the classification of idiopathic inflammatory myopathy: myositis-specific autoantibodies define useful homogeneous patient groups. Medicine (Baltimore). 1991; 70: 360–374.

Lundberg IE, Miller FW, Tajarnlund A, Bottal M. Diagnosis and classification of idiopathic inflammatory myopathies. J Intern Med. 2016; 280(1): 39–51.

Maeda MH. Idiopathic inflammatory myopathy and anti-aminoacyl-tRNA synthetase antibody. Brain Nerve. 2018; 70(4): 439–448.

Mahler M, Miller FW, Fritzler MJ. Idiopathic inflammatory myopathies and the anti-synthetase syndrome: a comprehensive review. Autoimmune Rev. 2014; 13: 367–371.

Marie I, Hatron PY, Dominique S, Cherin P, Mouthon L, Menard JF, et al. Short-term and long-term outcome of anti-Jo1-positive patients with anti-Ro52 antibody. Semin Arthritis Rheum. 2012; 41(6): 890–899.

Mescam-Mancini L, Allenbach Y, Hervier B, Devilliers H, et al. Anti-Jo-1 antibody-positive patients show a characteristic necrotizing perifascicular myositis. Brain. 2015: 2485–2492.

Patil AK, Prabhaker AT, Sivadasan A, Alexander M, et al. An usual case of inflammatory necrotizing myopathy and neuropathy with Pipestem capillaries. Neurol India. 2015: 63(1): 72–76.

Pestronk A. Acquired immune and inflammatory myopathies: pathologic classification. Curr Opin Rheumatol. 2011; 23: 595–604.

Pluk H, van Hoeve BJ, van Dooren SH, Stammen-Vogelzangs J, van der Heijden A, Schelhaas HJ, et al. Autoantibodies to cytosolic 5'-nucleotidase 1A in inclusion body myositis. Ann Neurol. 2013; 73(3): 397–407.

Rider LG, Miller FW. Deciphering the clinical presentations, pathogenesis, and treatment of the idiopathic inflammatory myopathies. JAMA. 2011; 12: 183–190.

Rinnenthal JL, Goebel HH, Preube C, et al. Inflammatory myopathy with abundant macrophages (IMAM): the immunology revisited. Neuromuscul Disord. 2014; 24(2): 151–155.

Satoh M, Tanaka S, Ceribelll A, Callse SJ, Chan EKL. A comprehensive overview on myositis-specific antibodies: new and old biomarkers in idiopathic inflammatory myopathy. Clin Rev Allergy Immunol. 2017; 52(1): 1–19.

Schmidt J. Current classification and management of inflammatory myopathies. J Neuromuscul Dis. 2018; 5(2): 109–129.

Schroder NW, Goebel HH, Brandis A, Ladhoff AM, Heppner FL, et al. Capillaries in necrotizing myopathy revisited. Neuromuscul Disord. 2013; 23(1): 66–74.

Senecal JL, Raynauld JP, Troyanov Y. Editorial: a new classification of adult autoimmune myositis. Arthritis Rheumatol. 2017; 69(5): 878–884.

Stenzel W, Goebel HH, Aronica E. Review: immune-mediated necrotizing myopathies–a heterogeneous group of diseases with specific myopathological features. Neuropathol Appl Neurobiol. 2012; 38: 632–646.

Sun Y, Liu Y, Yan B, Shi G. Interstitial lung disease in clinically amyopathic dermatomyositis (CADM) patients: a retrospective study of 41 Chinese Han patients. Rheumatol Int. 2013; 33(5): 1295–1302.

Targoff IN, Johnson AE, Miller FW. Antibody to signal recognition particle in polymyositis. Arthritis Rheum. 1990; 138: 3219–3223.

Targoff IN, Mamyrova G, Trieu EP, et al. A novel autoantibody to a 155-kD protein is associated with dermatomyositis. Arthritis Rheum. 2006; 54: 3682–3689.

Targoff IN. Update on myositis-specific and myositis-associated autoantibodies. Curr Opin Rheumatol. 2000; 12: 475–481.

Troyanov Y, Targoff IN, Tremblay JL, Goulet JR, Raymond Y, Senecal JL. Novel classification of idiopathic inflammatory myopathies based on overlap syndrome features and autoantibodies: analysis of 100 French Canadian patients. Medicine (Baltimore). 2005; 84: 231–249.

Uruha A, Nishikawa A, Tsuburaya RS, Hamanaka K, Kuwana M, Watanabe Y, et al. Sarcoplasmic MxA expression: a valuable marker of dermatomyositis. Neurology. 2017; 88(5): 493–500.

Uruha A, Suzuki S, Suzuki N, Nishino I. Perifascicular necrosis in anti-synthetase syndrome beyond anti-Jo-1. Brain. 2016; 139: e50.

Van de Vlekkert J, Hoogendijk JE, de Visser M. Myositis with endomysial cell invasion indicates inclusion body myositis even if other criteria are not fulfilled. Neuromuscul Disord. 2015; 25(6): 451–456.

Van der Meulen MFG, Bronner IM, Hoogendijk JE, Burger H, van Venrooij WJ, et al. Polymyositis – an overdiagnosed entity. Neurology. 2003; 61(3): 316–321.

CHAPTER 21

CHRONIC DENERVATION MYOPATHY

Ahmed Bamaga MD and Maher Kurdi MD

Contents

Long-standing neurogenic disease may result in denervation of the target musculature. This is rare in clinical practice and usually referred to as *chronic denervation myopathy*. The spectrum of potential causes ranges from hereditary or sporadic genetic mutations to neurodegenerative, inflammatory, and neoplastic processes. In addition, aging of muscle and some metabolic conditions are also accompanied by neuropathy. The most common sporadic or hereditary cause is anterior horn cell degeneration of the central nervous system. Amyotrophic lateral sclerosis (ALS) in adulthood and spinal muscular atrophy (SMA) in childhood are the best examples of denervation myopathies. Secondary acquired causes include any disease with severe peripheral neuropathy, due to any cause, affecting the innervated muscle. Table 21.1 lists the common denervation diseases in muscle pathology practice.

21.1 Chronic Denervation Atrophy (CDA)

CDA includes any neurological disease affecting the muscle, such as ALS, SMA, amyloidosis, and other axonal or demyelinating diseases.

Detailed clinical history and electrophysiological studies with nerve biopsy are required, particularly when the muscle biopsy is inconclusive. Some muscle biopsies show unequivocal changes while other biopsies are difficult to distinguish denervation atrophy from pseudomyopathy or muscular dystrophy (Figure 21.1a–c). Multiple internal nuclei, endomysial and perimysial fibrosis, regenerated muscle fibers, and selective type I atrophy are common features seen in muscular dystrophy rather than CDA.

Early-stage chronic denervation is characterized by loss of checkerboard pattern and scattered angulated fibers, highlighted with esterase and NADH stains. In SMA, these angulated fibers are replaced by the rounded shape

Table 21.1 Chronic denervation myopathic diseases.

Disease	Pattern	Cause	Clinical features	Investigation	Microscopic features
Chronic denervation atrophy	Hereditary acquired	Neuromyopathic change results from long-standing chronic denervation. Variants: • Early stage denervation • Partial denervation atrophy • Denervation with reinnervation • Severe denervation atrophy **Some cases are associated with myopathic change.	• Adult onset • Progressive distal and proximal weakness • Peripheral numbness • Fatigability • Fasciculation • Areflexia	CK is normal EMG/NCT: neuropathic	• Marked variation in fiber size • Loss of checkerboard pattern **Early stage:** • Type II > I atrophy • Type I fiber predominance • Angulated fibers (+) for esterase and NADH **Partial or severe stage:** • Several angulated fibers • Pyknotic nuclear clumps • Large or small fiber group atrophy • Fiber type grouping • Few cores and whorling fibers • Perimysial fibrosis • Degenerated fibers (red/pale) • Reinnervating fibers (target or targetoid fibers and hypertrophic fibers) <u>EM</u>: Group atrophy-myelin figures-none myelinated nerves—motor end plate empty

| Congenital hypomyelinating neuropathy | ARD ADD | **Type I:** MPZ gene mutation on Ch.1q23 encodes P0-protein. Allelic with CMTS-III **Type II:** EGR-2 gene mutation on Ch.10q21.3 encodes early growth response protein. Allelic with CMTS-1D/4 | • Early onset • Could be asymptomatic • Generalized hypotonic • Generalized weakness • Facial weakness • Absent reflexes • Arthrogryposis | CK is normal EMG: normal NCT: Severe demyelinating CSF: high protein | • Minimal variation in fiber size • Predominant type I atrophy • Denervation change • Absent fiber group atrophy **Nerve changes:** • Giant axons or axonal loss • Regenerating clusters • Onion bulb appearance |

Abbreviations: ADD: autosomal dominant disease. ARD: autosomal recessive, disease. CK: creatinine kinase. EMG: electromyography. NCT: nerve conduction test. EM: electron microscopy. MPZ: P0 protein. EGR-2: early growth response-2. CMTS: Charcot–Marie–Tooth syndrome. CSF: cerebrospinal fluid.

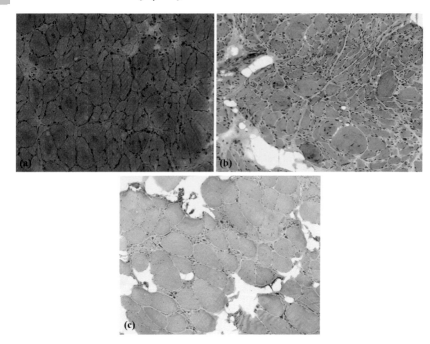

Figure 21.1 Histological differences between chronic denervation atrophy (CDA) and muscular atrophy (MD). **(a, b)** H&E sections from patients with CDA showing selective fiber atrophy and scattered target fibers. **(c)** H&E sections from a patient with MD show atrophic and hypertrophic fibers with multiple internal nuclei and pyknotic nuclear clumps. ×25.

of atrophic fibers. Unfortunately, these minimal neuropathic features are sometimes interpreted by non-expert pathologists as non-specific findings. However, clinical correlation is important in these cases. Partial or severe denervation is characterized by marked neuropathic features in the form of several angulated fibers, fiber type grouping, selective fiber trophy, few cores, and muscle fiber whorling (**Figure 21.2**). Fibers supplied by a single motor nerve will obviously not show atrophy, but compensatory hypertrophy may occur. The diagnosis of denervation should not be made unless the atrophy involves both muscle fiber types. In rare cases, denervating muscle fibers may lose their glycogen composition.

To date, there is no specific marker to distinguish atrophic fibers from real denervating fibers. Non-specific esterase can be used as an immunolabelling marker to highlight denervated fibers with brown-orange discoloration. The most characteristic features of the re-innervation process in muscle biopsy are hypertrophic fibers and target or targetoid fibers (**Figure 21.2a, e**).

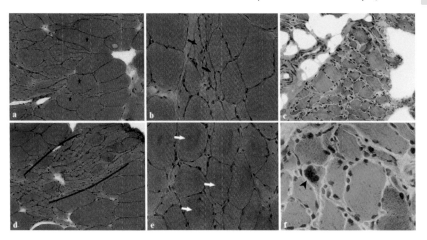

Figure 21.2 Histopathological features of chronic denervation atrophy. **(a)** Hypertrophic fibers (*). **(b)** Atrophic angulated fibers (*black arrows*). **(c)** Fiber-type grouping. **(d)** Selective fibers atrophy between two lines. **(e)** Target fibers (*white arrows*). **(f)** Pyknotic nuclear clumps. Different magnifications (×25−×40).

It is very difficult to distinguish CDA due to sporadic ALS from peripheral neuropathies due to chronic inflammatory demyelinating neuropathy (CIDP). CIDP affects the muscles when the condition is very severe. Nerve biopsy and electron microscopy can help to detect demyelinating features of the disease. In these cases, clinical correlation and additional laboratory investigating are advised.

Congenital hypomyelinating neuropathy (CHN) is a variant of chronic denervation myopathy with birth onset. It is clinically characterized by generalized hypotonia and weakness. In muscle biopsy, predominant type I atrophy with denervation change is the most common histological finding.

Amyloid neuropathy, another rare entity, has been explained in *Chapter 19*. It usually affects peripheral nerves and commonly progresses to involve the targeted musculature. The patient may present with neuropathic features that end in chronic denervation atrophy. Ultrastructural examination is important in these cases.

21.2 Spinal Muscular Atrophy (SMA)

Spinal muscular atrophy (SMA) is an autosomal recessive inherited neuromuscular disease characterized by degeneration of spinal cord motor neurons. It is caused by homozygous mutations of survival motor neuron 1 (SMN1) gene on both copies of chromosome 5q. The presence of a human unique SMN2 as a backup

Table 21.2 Classification of spinal muscular atrophy (SMA).

SMA type	Onset	SMN2 copies	Highest function	Survival rate
Type 0	Prenatal	1	Respiratory support	< 1 month
Type I: Werdnig Hoffman disease	0–6 months	2	Never able to sit	< 2 years
Type II: Dubowitz Syndrome	< 18 months	3–4	Never able to stand	> 2 years
Type III: Kugelberg–Welander Syndrome	> 18 months	3–4	Stand alone	Adult
Type IV	> 21 years	4–8	Stand alone	Adult

gene provides partially functional SMN protein and affects the severity of the phenotype. SMA was originally described in two infant brothers by Guido Werdnig in 1891 and in seven additional cases by Johan Hoffmann from 1893 to 1900. The International Consortium on SPA sponsored by the Muscular Dystrophy Association in 1991 suggested phenotype classification of SMA based on the highest level of motor function and age of onset (**Table 21.2**). Subsequent modifications added a type I for adult-onset cases and included a type 0 for patients with prenatal onset and death within weeks.

Patients usually experience progressive muscular atrophy and weakness. Cognition and intellect are not affected. Many affected patients are born with floppy baby syndrome, whereas adult cases may have better motor function. SMA used to be diagnosed by muscle biopsy that typically shows denervation atrophy; in particular, features of group atrophy, hypertrophied type 1 fibers, and small fibers either mixed or type 2 (**Figure 21.3**). Muscle biopsy is done only for diagnostic exclusion of SMA and is not used as a confirmatory tool. Genetic testing looking for SMN1 deletion widely replaced the muscle biopsy. Because the disease is associated with poor outcomes, multidisciplinary management of different care supports is required.

Several different approaches have been utilized to treat SMA. The first is splicing modification of SMN2 in order to improve protein production. Developed by Biogen, Spinraza (nusinersen) is the first Food and Drug Administration (FDA) approved medication for SMA treatment. It is an

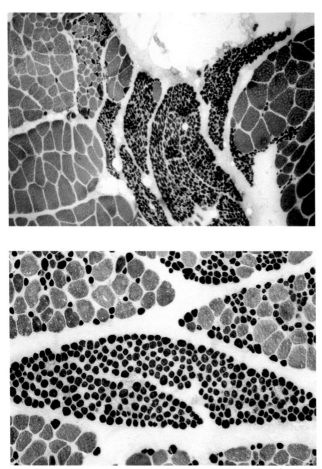

Figure 21.3 Sections from patient with SMA, stained with ATPase 9.4, show atrophy of both fiber types. Most of the larger fibers are type 1 and many of the atrophic fibers appear as type 2 fibers. (×10). This figure was published in Muscle biopsy: A practical approach, Chapter 9, V. Dubowitz, Neurogenic diseases, Page 245, Copyright Elsevier 2013.

antisense oligonucleotide targeted to SMN2 pre-messenger RNA (pre-mRNA) that increases the proportion of SMN2 mRNA transcripts that include exon 7. This will let the body produce more SMN proteins. The second approach is the replacement of the SMN1 gene. Gene therapy for SMA is the most advanced medical approach that directly targets the dysfunctional SMN1 gene. Zolgensma (onasemnogene abeparvovec-xioi) is the second FDA approved medication given for children less than 2 years of age with bi-allelic mutations in SMN1 genes. It is an adeno-associated virus vector-based gene therapy.

In summary, chronic denervation myopathy is a challenging condition in clinical practice that requires clinical correlation and careful interpretation of nerve and muscle biopsy. The diagnosis is always not established through histopathology; additional laboratory tests and EM are helpful.

References

Dubowitz V. Chaos in classification of the spinal muscular atrophies of childhood. Neuromuscul Disord. 1991; 1: 77–80.

Dubowitz V. Pathology of experimentally re-innervated skeletal muscle. J Neurol Neurosurg Psychiatr. 1967; 30: 99–110.

Harati Y, Butler IJ. Congenital hypomyelinating neuropathy. J Neurol Neurosurg Psych. 1985; 48: 1269–1276.

Kochanski A, Drac H, Kabzinska D, Ryniewicz B, et al. A novel MPZ gene mutation in congenital neuropathy with hypomyelination. Neurology. 2004; 62: 2122–2123.

Lunn MR, Wang CH. Spinal muscular atrophy. Lancet. 2008; 371: 2120–2133.

Schorling D, Pechmann A, Kirschner J. Advances in treatment of spinal muscular atrophy- new phenotypes, new challenges, new implications for care. J Neuromuscul Dis. 2020; 7(1): 1–13.

Sugarman EA, Nagan N, Zhu H, Akmaev VR, et al. Pan-ethnic carrier screening and prenatal diagnosis for spinal muscular atrophy: clinical laboratory analysis of > 72,400 specimens. Eur J Hum Genet. 2012; 20(1): 27–32.

Wang CH, Finkel RS, Bertini E, Schroth M, et al. Consensus statement for standard of care in spinal muscular atrophy. J Child Neurol. 2007; 22(8): 1027–1049.

CHAPTER 22

AXIAL MYOPATHY

Axial myopathy is a rare neuromuscular disease entity affecting paraspinal musculature. It is characterized by progressive weakness of spinal extensor muscles. It could be predominant constituting the major part of myopathy or widespread to involve other skeletal muscles. It can also be a separate condition (myopathy with predominant axial involvement) or a part of other myopathic dystrophy diseases.

The most common clinical characteristic feature is abnormal posture, most notably camptocormia, also known as bent spine. Spinal rigidity is a common associated feature. Physical examination of neck mobility, muscle strength, and electrodiagnostic testing are important assessments to confirm the abnormal pattern seen in the paraspinal muscles. Fatty replacement of paraspinal muscle is commonly seen in magnetic resonance imaging (**Figure 22.1**).

In muscle biopsy, normal paraspinal muscle histologically mimics myopathy. Moth-eaten fibers, cores, splitting fibers, fiber-type grouping, and mitochondrial changes all can be seen in normal paraspinal muscles. These features make the diagnosis very difficult to reach. However, the surgeon or clinician should know exactly which muscle must be biopsied. Clinical correlation is also recommended to confirm the myopathic presentation of the disease.

Axial myopathy can be classified into two major variants:

1. Myopathy with predominant axial involvement
2. Axial myopathy as part of other myopathic diseases

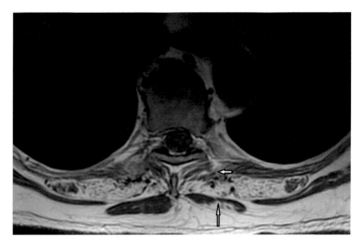

Figure 22.1 An axial T1-MRI of a 34-year-old man shows fatty replacement of paraspinal muscle (*white arrows*).

The most well-known diseases predominantly affecting axial muscles are selenoprotein deficiency due to SNP1 and lamin A/C gene mutations. Heterozygous mutations in the skeletal muscle (RYR-1) that encode Ryanodine receptor-1 have recently been recognized as a rare novel entity associated with predominant axial myopathy. It is a late-onset condition associated with bent spine syndrome, camptocormia, proximal weakness, and lordosis. Pathologically, it is characterized by myopathic features, scattered cores, desmin aggregation, and mitochondrial abnormalities (**Figure 22.2**).

GSD-II (Pompe disease) and GSD-V (McArdle's disease) also reported pronounced paraspinal muscle involvement. Inclusion body myositis, mitochondrial myopathy, Duchenne muscular dystrophy, FHMD, Bethlem myopathy, calpainopathy, myotonic dystrophy, and MHY-7-related myopathy also showed some paraspinal muscle involvement.

In summary, paraspinal muscle in myopathy may show pathology even if muscle biopsy is normal. Because of the co-existing features of normal and abnormal findings in axial muscles, muscle biopsies in the clinical evaluation of axial myopathy collectively are not recommended.

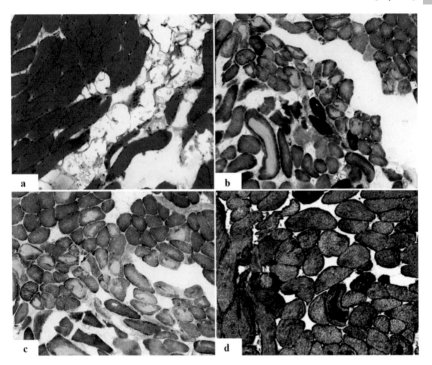

Figure 22.2 Histological features of axial myopathy with RYR-1 gene mutation in a 65-year-old woman presenting with camptocormia. **(a)** Fatty infiltration to muscle fibers with minimal myopathic change. **(b)** Multiple irregular cores seen on SDH stain. **(c)** COX-negative fibers with multiple cores seen through combined COX-SDH stain. **(d)** Desmin aggregation inside the cores. ×20.

References

Chemla JC, Kanter RJ, Carboni MP, Smith EC. Two children with "dropped head" syndrome due to Lamin A/C mutations. Muscle Nerve. 2010; 42: 839–841.

Dahlqvist JR, Vissing CR, Thomsen C, Vissing J. Severe paraspinal muscle involvement in facioscapulohumeral muscular dystrophy. Neurology. 2014; 83: 1178–1183.

Delcey V, Hachulla E, Michon-Pasturel U, et al. Camptocormia: a sign of axial myopathy. Report of 7 cases. Rev Med Interne. 2002; 23(2): 144–154.

Gomez-Puerta JA, Peris P, Grau JM, Martinez MA, Guanabens N. Camptocormia as a clinical manifestation of mitochondrial myopathy. Clin Rheumatol. 2007; 26: 1017–1019.

Goodman BP, Liewluck T, Crum BA, Spinner RJ. Camptocormia due to inclusion body myositis. J Clin Neuromuscul Dis. 2012; 14: 78–81.

Kocaaga Z, Bal S, Turan Y, Gurgan A, Esmeli F. Camptocormia and dropped head syndrome as a clinic picture of myotonic myopathy. Joint Bone Spine. 2008; 75: 730–733.

Laforet P, Doppler V, Caillaud C, Laloui K, Claeys KG, et al. Rigid spine syndrome revealing late-onset Pompe disease. Neuromuscul Disord. 2010; 20: 128–130.

Loseth S, Voermans NC, Torbergsen T, Lillis S, et al. A novel late-onset axial myopathy associated with mutation in the skeletal muscle ryanodine receptor (RYR1) gene. J Neurol. 2013; 260(6): 1504–1510.

Park JM, Kim YJ, Yoo JH, Hong YB, Park JH, Koo H, et al. A novel MYH7 mutation with prominent paraspinal and proximal muscle involvement. Neuromuscul Disord. 2013; 23: 580–586.

Sakiyama Y, Okamoto Y, Higuchi I, Inamori Y, et al. A new phenotype of mitochondrial disease characterized by familial late-onset predominant axial myopathy and encephalopathy. Acta Neuropathol. 2011; 121: 775–783.

Witting N, Andersen LK, Vissing J. Axial myopathy: an overlooked feature of muscle disease. Brain. 2016; 139: 13–22.

Witting N, Duno M, Piraud M, Vissing J. Severe axial myopathy in McArdle disease. JAMA Neurol. 2014; 71: 88–90.

CHAPTER 23

FASCIITIS

Fasciitis is an acute inflammatory disease of the fascia, either due to immune-mediated reaction or acquired by intramuscular vaccinations. The inflammation is localized to the fascia and rarely infiltrates into the muscle fibers. However, perimysial inflammation is always present and associated with lymphohistiocytic infiltrates. Careful clinical history and laboratory investigations may help the clinician to reach the diagnosis. Muscle biopsy in these cases is performed to rule out any abnormal myopathic or neuropathic conditions.

Table 23.1 summarizes the subtypes of fasciitis that are commonly seen in clinicopathological practice.

Eosinophilic fasciitis (EF) is a rare scleroderma-like syndrome of unknown etiology categorized as an immune-allergic disorder. It is clinically characterized by painful skin indurations, hypereosinophilia, hypergammaglobinemia, and elevated erythrocyte sedimentation rate (ESR). The disease can be associated with several inflammatory and immunological disorders such as scleroderma, systemic sclerosis, and lymphoma. The most characteristic clinical feature is localized painful swelling or mass. Full-thickness wedge biopsy of the affected skin may show a localized lymphoplasmacytic inflammation with abundant macrophages. The lymphocytes are mainly CD8 cytotoxic T-cells.

Other associated histological features include prominent eosinophilia, perimysial inflammation, and perifascicular atrophy. Necrotizing granuloma are occasionally seen in the biopsy. The condition should be distinguished from the perimysial inflammation called perimyositis.

Macrophagic myofasciitis is due to the persistence of vaccine-derived aluminum hydroxide at the site of intramuscular injection. It is usually associated with hepatitis A or B and tetanus vaccines. The affected child

Table 23.1 Subtypes of fasciitis.

Disease	Pattern	Cause	Clinical features	Investigation	Microscopic features

Eosinophilic fasciitis (Shulman disease)	Immune mediated	Scleroderma-like syndrome with unknown cause, associated with eosinophilic toxic proteins and mast cell degranulation Should be differentiated from perimyositis	• Adult onset
			• Fever
			• Myalgia
			• Painful skin mass
			• Can be associated with: lymphoma and nivolumab drug
				CK is normal
				IgG is ↑
				Eosinophilia
				EMG: myopathic
				MRI: T2 signal in fascia or muscle
					• Subcutaneous inflammation associated with:
					  a. Lymphoplasmacytic cells (CD8+ CD138+)
					  b. Abundant macrophages (CD68+)
					  c. Prominent eosinophils
					• Occasional granuloma
					• Perimysial inflammation
					• Perifascicular atrophy (rare)

Macrophagic myofasciitis	Acquired	Immune-mediated reaction post-vaccination causes intramuscular accumulation of macrophages containing vaccine-derived aluminum hydroxide Common vaccines: hepatitis B, tetanus, and hepatitis A	• Adult onset • Common in French • Fever and rash • Myalgia • Focal weakness • Can be associated with CNS motor symptoms	CK is normal CRP is ↑ EMG: normal CSF: high protein	• Normal muscle appearance • Macrophage aggregation in perimysium • Aluminum deposits • PAS (+) inclusions • Absent MNGC <u>EM:</u> Macrophage containing aluminum crystals

Abbreviations: CK: creatinine kinase. EMG: electromyography. IgG: immunoglobulin G. MRI: magnetic resonance imaging. CRP: C-reactive protein. CSF: cerebrospinal fluid. MNGC: multinucleated giant cells.

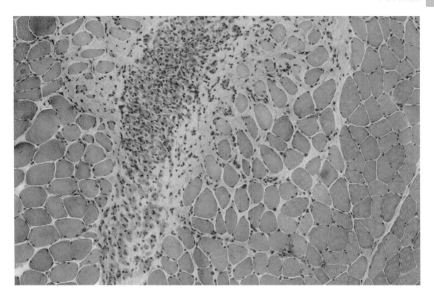

Figure 23.1 H&E section from a patient with macrophagic fasciitis. There is extensive extrafascicular inflammation of macrophages. This figure was published in Muscle biopsy: A practical approach, Chapter 23, V. Dubowitz, Neurogenic diseases, Page 547, Copyright Elsevier 2013.

presents with fever, myalgia, focal skin swelling, and other associated vaccination side effects. Blood work and electrodiagnostic tests usually show non-specific findings. Histologically, the muscle fibers look normal but there is a diffuse infiltration of CD68+ macrophages through the perimysium, without any structural damage to the muscle fibers (**Figure 23.1**). PAS (+) inclusions containing aluminum deposits may sometimes be seen. Ultrastructurally, aluminum crystalloid materials are seen inside the macrophages.

References

Mazori DR, Femia AN, Vleugels RA. Eosinophilic fasciitis: an update review on diagnosis and treatment. Curr Rheumatol Rep. 2017; 19(12): 74.

Onajin O, Wieland CN, Peters MS, Lohse CM, Lehman JS. Clinicopathologic and immunophenotypic features of eosinophilic fasciitis and morphea profunda: a comparative study of 27 cases. J Am Acad Dermatol. 2018; 68(1): 121–128.

Soares Santos D, Santos A, Rebelo O, Santos RM. Macrophagic myofasciitis: a challenging diagnosis. BMJ Case Rep. 2018; bcr2018224602.

PART III
NERVE

CHAPTER 24
CLASSIFICATION OF NEUROPATHY

Peripheral neuropathy is a general medical term describing diseases affecting peripheral nerves. It may affect sensory nerves causing sensory neuropathy or motor nerves causing motor neuropathy. Coexisting motor and sensory disturbances are called sensorimotor neuropathy.

Neuropathy may also affect one nerve (mononeuropathy) or multiple nerves (polyneuropathy). The term *mononeuritis multiplex* is applied when one or more separate nerves in disparate areas are affected. Mononeuropathy should be distinguished clinically from polyneuropathy as mono-type usually occurs as result of local injury or focal disease. Polyneuropathy is a common condition that occurs in almost all neurological diseases.

There are several ways to classify neuropathies. They can be classified according to the number, distribution, and types of nerves affected, or they can be categorized based on the underlying causative mechanism. However, neuropathies are best classified, by the pathological pattern, into axonal neuropathy and demyelinating neuropathy. Each group may be subcategorized into hereditary or acquired variants based on the underlying pathogenic mechanism. Both groups may contain some histopathological features from the opposite groups. For example, paraproteinemic neuropathy may show axonal degeneration and segmental demyelination as primary pathology.

Neuropathy may also progress to affect the muscle, in a new term called *neuromyopathy*. It is uncommon that myopathy causes secondary neuropathic disease. This is completely dependent on the underlying pathology.

Classification of Neuropathy

The best method to diagnose neuropathy clinically is electrodiagnostic studies such as nerve conduction test (NCT). NCT helps clinicians and pathologists understand which pattern of neuropathy exists. NCT also aids in minimizing the differential diagnosis. The need for nerve biopsy is also rare in clinical practice. This is because nerve biopsies carry low sensitivity in the diagnosis. Clinicians may order nerve biopsy for the following reasons: (1) progressive disease without improvement on current treatment, (2) expected hereditary cause, or (3) assessment of the disease progression or remission. Nevertheless, some practitioners ask for nerve biopsy as a routine test when the clinical investigations show no clinical answer. The interpretation of nerve biopsy should always be with clinical correlation to avoid any error in the diagnosis.

As we mentioned before, neuropathies are classified pathologically into axonal-type (associated with axonal degeneration) or demyelinating type (associated with segmental demyelination) (**Figure 24.1**).

Axonal neuropathy is subcategorized into acquired and hereditary spectrums. The most common cause of acquired axonal neuropathy is long-standing uncontrolled diabetes (see *Chapter 30*). Although hereditary conditions are rare, Charcot–Marie–Tooth disease (CMTD) is considered at the top of the differential diagnosis.

On the other hand, demyelinating neuropathy is subdivided into two variants: acquired/secondary versus hereditary/autoimmune. The most common cause of acquired demyelinating neuropathy is marked axonal degeneration (see *Chapter 27*). For the immune-mediated spectrum, acute and chronic inflammatory demyelinating diseases (ACDN/CIDN) are considered the most common cause of inflammatory demyelinating neuropathy. These two patterns of neuropathies (axonal versus demyelinating) are sometimes difficult to distinguish by only electrodiagnostic tests and nerve biopsy. Multidisciplinary approaches using clinical, laboratory, and genetic testing are required.

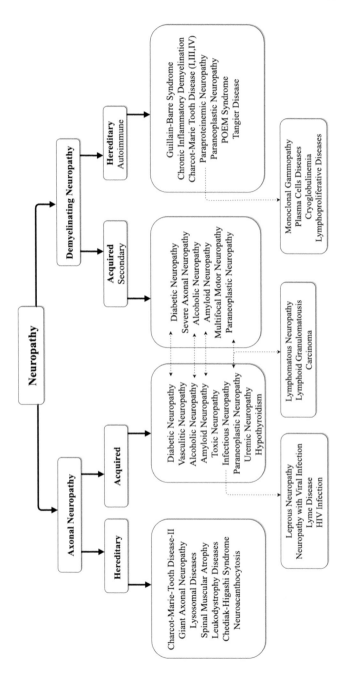

Figure 24.1 Classification of peripheral neuropathy.

References

Hughes RAC. Peripheral neuropathy. BMJ. 2002; 324: 466–469.

Reilly MM. Classification of the hereditary motor and sensory neuropathies. Curr Opin Neurol. 2000; 13: 561–564.

Rosenberg NR, Portegies P, de Visser M, Vermeulen M. Diagnostic investigation of patients with chronic polyneuropathy: evaluation of a clinical guideline. J Neurol Neurosurg Psychiatry. 2001; 71: 205–209.

CHAPTER 25

DIAGNOSTIC APPROACH IN NERVE BIOPSY

Microscopic inspection of nerve biopsy tissue requires clinical and pathological correlation. Electrodiagnostic tests usually direct pathologists to the correct track to follow. Because histological changes are sometimes subtle, pathologists should follow a systematic approach to evaluate abnormal findings seen in biopsy (**Figure 25.1**). Indeed, relating the pathology to the clinical picture is paramount to diagnosis.

Epoxy-embedded thick sections treated with toluidine stain are the best tool to evaluate nerve biopsy. This technique was discussed in *Chapter 6*. Some institutions use hematoxylin and eosin (H&E) stain or H&E with Luxol fast blue (LFB) for microscopic evaluation. The essential set for nerve biopsy must include sections treated with H&E, toluidine, and neurofilament stains. Pathologists should have the impression of the nerve biopsy finding from lower magnification. Tissue examination should begin from the external epineurial layer and then go deeply to the perineurium and endoneurium. Artifactual distortion is a common problem in any nerve tissue processing and must be carefully interpreted to avoid any misdiagnosis.

Partial or complete loss of myelinated fibers may be associated with primary demyelination or axonal degeneration with secondary demyelination. This is considered a diagnostic challenge when it becomes difficult to distinguish primary from secondary demyelination (see *Chapter 27*). The presence of myelin ovoids and myelin figures with ultrastructural contents of degenerated axons suggests axonal neuropathy rather than demyelinating neuropathy. Acute presentation of axonal neuropathy usually occurs within a week and is associated with focal traumatic injury. Chronic axonal neuropathy is defined as long-standing degeneration of the axons, which is occasionally associated with minimal demyelination.

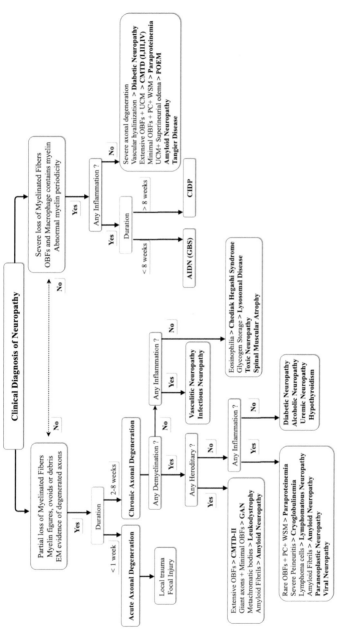

Figure 25.1 Diagnostic approach of neuropathy through nerve biopsy. OBFs: onion-bulb formations. CMTD: Charcot–Marie–Tooth disease. GAN: giant axonal neuropathy. WSM: widely spaced myelin. PC: plasma cells. AIDN: acute inflammatory demyelinating neuropathy. CIDN: chronic inflammatory demyelinating neuropathy. GBS: Guillain–Barre syndrome. UCM: uncompacted myelin. POEM: polyneuropathy, organomegaly, endocrinopathy, monoclonal gammopathy, and skin changes.

There are two pathways:

1. **Axonal degeneration with minimal or no demyelination:**
   a. with inflammation such as vasculitic or infectious neuropathies
   b. without inflammation such as toxic neuropathy, spinal muscular atrophy, eosinophilia syndrome, and lysosomal diseases.

2. **Axonal degeneration with marked demyelination:**

   a. hereditary causes such as Charcot–Marie–Tooth disease (CMTD)-type II, giant axonal neuropathy (GAN), amyloid neuropathy, and, rarely, leukodystrophy. Onion-bulb formations characterize both CMTD and GAN due to the recurrent demyelination-remyelination process.
   b. non-hereditary causes with inflammation, such as paraproteinemic neuropathy, paraneoplastic process, and, rarely, viral-induced neuropathy. If inflammation is absent, diabetic neuropathy is the main cause in this category.

Inflammation types and sites differ from disease to disease. However, the inflammation is considered serious when it occurs in the perineurium or endoneurium. Perivascular inflammatory cuffs are sometimes non-specific. Types of inflammation can be distinguished using immunolabelling markers such as CD45 and CD68. Although paraproteinemia is associated with minimal inflammation, the diagnosis requires ultrastructural examination of EM sections.

Demyelinating neuropathy is clinically expected when electrodiagnostic testing shows predominant features of demyelination while the histopathology shows preserved axons. However, minimal axonal drop-outs have been observed in a few cases of primary demyelination.

There are two pathways:

1. **Demyelination with inflammation:** The most common condition in this category is acute or chronic inflammatory demyelinating neuropathies. Chronic-type is defined when clinical symptoms progress for more than 8 weeks or the acute-type undergoes remitting and relapsing ictus. The diagnosis of these two entities depends on several parameters including histological sections, immunohistochemistry, and ultrastructural examination; the latter shows abnormal periodicity of myelination.
2. **Demyelination with no evidence of inflammation:** This is commonly associated with marked axonal neuropathy when the disease progresses to affect the myelin sheaths. Neuropathy associated with long-standing non-controlled diabetes is another common cause under this category. EM sectioning is a useful diagnostic method to differentiate between types of non-inflammatory demyelinating diseases.

205

In conclusion, the nerve biopsy method is usually neither sensitive nor specific for the diagnosis. It is considered an additional test frequently used to rule out other neuropathies or to follow up on the remission and relapsing status of a particular disease. Total assessments of myelination, inflammation, and myelin periodicity are major parameters in the diagnostic approach.

CHAPTER 26
AXONAL NEUROPATHY

Axonal degeneration (AD) is clinically known as *axonal neuropathy*. It occurs when the axon of injured nerve fiber is separated from its original site (**Figure 26.1**). After injury, the axonal skeleton disintegrates, and the axonal membrane breaks apart. This process is usually followed by degradation of the myelin sheath and infiltration of macrophages. Calcium influx signaling promotes resealing of the injured site. Failure to deliver sufficient quantities of axonal protein, nicotinamide mononucleotide adenylyl transferase 2 (NMAT2), might be the cause behind this pathological event. Schwann cells immediately respond to this process by extrusion of their myelin sheaths and downregulation of myelin genes. If the distal end-sprouts are able to reach the injured site, the re-innervation process occurs in the form of regeneration. Failure to reach the injured site may cause secondary demyelination, which is sometimes mistaken as primary demyelination (see *Chapter 27*).

Axonal degeneration can be anterograde (Wallerian), retrograde (dying-back) or combined (**Figure 26.1**). Motor axons degenerate earlier than sensory axons. Wallerian-type degeneration constitutes the microscopic reactions of a nerve segment distal to a site of crush or transection injury. This is rare in clinical practice and commonly associated with ischemia or trauma.

Neuropathy resulting from degeneration of the distal parts of the axon with progression proximally toward the cell body is called dying-back neuropathy. It is the most common clinicopathological pattern seen in axonal polyneuropathy. Several theories have attempted to explain the pathologic mechanism. Unfortunately, the explanation was manifold and not backed by scientific evidence. However, the disease is clinically associated with several causes including diabetes, uremia, infection, amyloidosis, and alcohol (**Table 26.1**). Hereditary etiology was also reported. The most common

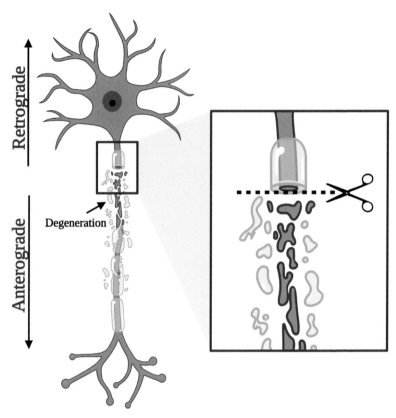

Figure 26.1 An illustrated diagram shows the two types of axonal degeneration. *This figure was created with Biorender.com.*

hereditary causes of dying-back neuropathy are Charcot–Marie–Tooth disease (CMTD) and giant axonal neuropathy (GAN).

Because dying-back degeneration always affects sensory fibers, the earliest manifestation will be stocking–glove symmetrical sensory neuropathy, and the histological pattern may show relatively more severe loss of large myelinated fibers. This is clearly identified in electrodiagnostic studies (see *Chapter 3*).

One of the best methods to examine AD is through epoxy-embedded toluidine sections. The histological features are dependent on the disease stage. Acute axonal degeneration is commonly characterized by myelin ovoids and axonal swelling. This process immediately occurs after the nerve injury. The hallmark feature of chronic type degeneration is partial or complete loss of myelin sheaths that surround the axons (**Figure 26.2a**). It is sometimes difficult to appreciate axonal degeneration in histological sections; however,

Table 26.1 Causes of axonal neuropathy.

Acquired	Hereditary
Diabetes	Charcot–Marie–Tooth disease
Uremia	Giant axonal neuropathy
Alcohol	Spinal muscular atrophy
Amyloidosis	Lysosomal diseases
Vasculitis	Adrenoleukodystrophy
Hypothyroidism	Porphyria cutanea tardia
Trauma	Chédiak-Higashi disease
Infection	Neuroacanthocytosis
Toxin	Xeroderma pigmentosum
Vitamin deficiency	Bassen-Kornzweig disease
Carcinomatosis	Unknown

ultrastructural examination is considered a golden confirmatory technique. In early stages, the myelin disintegrates and shrinks forming axoplasmic pallor or osmophilic materials. Later, the axoplasm turns dark and may contain lipid droplets. These are typically called myelin figures or debris. They are commonly accompanied with macrophages containing lipids, collagen pockets, and flattened Schwann cells (**Figure 26.3a–c**). Aggregated organelles, Schwann cell lipid droplets, absent axons, myeloid bodies, and tubulovesicular profiles in axoplasm are rarely seen. Mitochondrial abnormalities are other

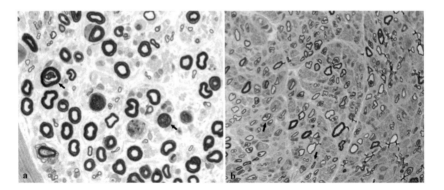

Figure 26.2 Toluidine sections from a patient with axonal neuropathy. **(a)** Section shows axonal degeneration with a partial loss of myelinated fibers, myelin figures, or ovoids (*red arrow*), and axonal swelling (*black arrow*). Reprinted with permission from Dr. Robert Hammond, Western University, Canada. **(b)** Section shows axonal regeneration with scattered thinly myelinated fibers and rare sprouts (*black arrows*).

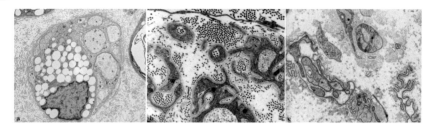

Figure 26.3 EM section shows ultrastructural features of axonal degeneration with regeneration. **(a)** Macrophage containing lipid droplets. **(b)** Collagen pockets. **(c)** Flattened Schwann cell basal laminae. Reprinted by permission from Springer Nature, Biopsy diagnosis of Peripheral Neuropathy, by Juan M. Bilbao and Robert E. Schmidt, 2nd ed Copyright, 2015.

rare findings and can be identified in vitamin E deficiency and some toxic neuropathies.

Unmyelinated fibers degenerate the same way as myelinated fibers degenerate, but it is very rare to see myelin ovoids with unmyelinated fiber degeneration. Remnants of large myelinated axons can also be seen throughout the section. The small axons are relatively preserved. Of the rare features, macrophages containing lipid debris inside the basal lamina of Schwann cells were also described. The most troublesome story is a biopsy that shows chronic axonal loss with a variable number of inappropriately thinly myelinated axons.

Every AD is followed by axonal regeneration, which starts within 2 days of the injury. Usually identified in late stage, the histological features are characterized by clusters of small thinly myelinated sheaths (**Figure 26.2b**) and regenerating sprouts (**Figure 26.4a,b**). These sprouts are groups of myelinated

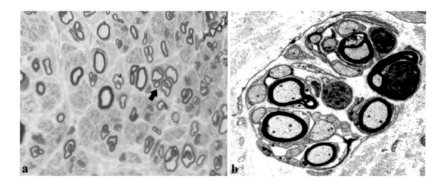

Figure 26.4 Regenerating sprouts indicate axonal regeneration. **(a)** Toluidine section. **(b)** EM section. Reprinted by permission from Springer Nature, Biopsy diagnosis of Peripheral Neuropathy, by Juan M. Bilbao and Robert E. Schmidt, 2nd ed Copyright, 2015.

Table 26.2 Pathological features of axonal degeneration and regeneration.

Pathology	Definition	Pathological findings
Axonal degeneration • Myelinated • Unmyelinated	**A**: Anterograde degeneration "*Wallerian*" Part of axon is separated from soma distal to site of injury **B**: Retrograde degeneration "*dying back*" Part of axon is separated from soma close to site of injury **C**: Dual type degeneration	**Acute**: Myelin ovoid-axonal swelling **Chronic**: Partial or complete loss of myelin, dark axoplasm, myelin containing lipids <u>EM</u>: Myelin figures, axonal pallor, macrophages, absent axons, flattened Schwann cells, collagen pockets, aggregated organelles, Schwann cell lipid droplets, TVP
Axonal regeneration	Regeneration of axons by Schwann cells within 2 days of axonal degeneration "about 3–5 mm/day"	Regenerating sprouts Thin myelin sheath Pseudo onion-bulb appearance <u>EM</u>: Regenerated sprouts, thin myelinated sheath, bands of Büngner

Abbreviations: EM: electron microscopy. TVP: tubulovesicular profiles.

and thinly unmyelinated fibers with complementary shape encircled basal lamina. Neurofilament stain can help to highlight the axonal growth by showing the filamentous elements in each fiber. Although thinly myelinated sheaths are common features in axonal regeneration, they are also remarkable features in the remyelination process. The only way to differentiate between them is through ultrastructural examination.

In EM, the hallmark feature of axonal regeneration is regenerating sprouts. It may be associated with tubulovesicular elements. Band of Büngner is another common finding. In some instances, failure of regeneration may occur and results in marked swelling of growth cones, lipid containing Schwann cells, and empty basal laminae.

Degenerated axons can also accompany some additional features of other neurological diseases. **Table 26.3** lists the uncommon pathological features affecting degenerated axons with their differential diagnoses.

Table 26.3 Differential diagnosis of uncommon axonal abnormalities.

Axonal abnormalities	Differential diagnosis
Giant axons	Acute AD, GAN, diabetic neuropathy, vitamin B12 deficiency, glue sniffing, amyloidosis, toxic neuropathy
Glycogenosomes	Diabetic neuropathy, hypothyroidism, lysosomal diseases
Polyglucosan bodies	Diabetic neuropathy, polyglucosan body disease, lysosomal diseases
Axonal atrophy	Friedreich's ataxia, cisplatin toxicity
Paracrystallin inclusions	GAN, Charcot–Marie–Tooth disease, Fabry disease

Abbreviations: AD: axonal degeneration. GAN: giant axonal neuropathy.

In summary, axonal degeneration and regeneration can be identified through nerve biopsy and electron microscopy. Every axonal degeneration is associated with secondary demyelination. It is actually difficult to specify the underlying cause only from histopathological assessment; however, clinicopathological correlation is recommended. In the coming chapters, we describe some common peripheral nerve diseases presenting with axonal degeneration. We highlight the common pathological features associated with them.

References

Chaudry V, Glass JD, Griffin JW. Wallerian degeneration in peripheral nerve disease. Neurol Clin. 1992; 10: 613–627.

Court FA, Midha R, Cisterna BA, et al. Morphological evidence for a transport of ribosomes from Schwann cells to regenerating axons. Glia. 2011; 59: 1529–1539.

Dyck PJ, Hopkins AP. Electron microscopic observations on degeneration and regeneration of unmyelinated fibres. Brain. 1972; 95: 223–234.

Gilley J, Coleman M. Endogenous NMNAT2 is an essential survival factor for maintenance of healthy axons. Plos Biology. 2010. 8(1): e1000300.

Schlaepfer WW, Hasler MB. Characterization of the calcium induced disruption of neurofilaments in rat peripheral nerves. Brain Res. 1979; 168: 299–309.

Wang JT, Medress ZA, Barres BA. Axon degeneration mechanisms of a self-destruction pathway. J Cell Biol. 2012; 196(1): 7–18.

CHAPTER 27

DEMYELINATING NEUROPATHY

Segmental demyelination is clinically known as *demyelinating neuropathy*. It is characterized by focal degeneration of myelin sheath with axonal sparing. In rare and severe cases, the axons may be affected and accompanied with axonal degeneration. Demyelination mechanically occurs either due to macrophage antibody-mediated attack or marked axonal atrophy. It should be determined whether the process is fundamentally axonal or demyelinating, as this will affect the treatment and prognosis. Electrodiagnostic tests can occasionally distinguish axonal degeneration from demyelination but will not specify the type of demyelination. The distinction is usually not obvious as Schwann cells and axons are interdependent. As we described in the previous chapter, axonal degeneration can be followed by secondary demyelination. Pathologists must distinguish this type of demyelination through histopathological and ultrastructural examinations. Bear in mind that in primary demyelination, the axons are always preserved.

Primary demyelination occurs as a consequence of Schwann cell metabolism defect with inability to maintain the myelin sheath. It may also result from a direct attack on myelin. **Table 27.1** summarizes the general pathological causes of primary and secondary demyelination.

The characteristic features of demyelination in nerve biopsy are categorized based on the process activity. In early stage of active demyelination. Schwann cell vacuolation, macrophage accumulation, and myeloid bodies are seen. Small myelin ovoids are scattered within the section, which indicate ongoing degeneration. These ovoids cannot be distinguished from the ones seen in the acute axonal degeneration process in which myelination is damaged. Partial or complete loss of myelination surrounding the axons with myelin debris-filled macrophages is the hallmark feature of demyelination (**Figure 27.1a**) (**Table 27.2**). In some cases, perivascular or endoneurial inflammation is seen. The inflammation mainly consists of macrophages and scattered lymphocytes. The most common cause

Table 27.1 Causes of primary and secondary demyelinating neuropathy.

Primary "autoimmune/hereditary"	Secondary "acquired"
AIDP	Severe axonal neuropathy
CIDP	Diabetic neuropathy
CMTD "HMSN"	Multiple myeloma
Paraproteinemia	Paraproteinemia
Macroglobulinemia	Thiamine deficiency
Multifocal motor neuropathy	Alcohol
Lymphoma	Multifocal motor neuropathy
Leukodystrophy	Paraneoplastic neuropathy
POEM	
Tangier disease	

Abbreviations: AIDP: acute Inflammatory demyelinating polyneuropathy. CIDP: chronic inflammatory demyelinating polyneuropathy. POEM: polyneuropathy, organomegaly, endocrinopathy, monoclonal gammopathy, and skin changes. CMTD: Charcot–Marie–Tooth disease. HMSN: hereditary motor sensory neuropathy.

of demyelinating neuropathy associated with inflammation is acute and chronic inflammatory demyelinating polyneuropathy (ACDP/CIDP).

Distinguishing primary demyelination from secondary demyelination has proven difficult. Axonal dropouts are commonly associated with secondary demyelination while axons are preserved in primary demyelination. Neurofilament stain helps to highlight the preserved axons and filamentous component of the fibers. Numerous thinly myelinated axons with few axonal dropouts suggest primary demyelination. The presence of thinly myelinated axons with significant axonal loss suggests secondary demyelination or incomplete regeneration.

Electron microscopic examination is considered very helpful to distinguish primary from secondary type as it studies the exact pathology of myelin and axons.

Demyelination may sometimes be accompanied by remyelination (**Figure 27.1c**). This process is characterized histologically with the presence of thinly myelinated fibers or Remak fibers. It is difficult to distinguish axonal regeneration from remyelination unless the disease is axonal type, or the axons are histologically preserved. The hallmark sign of recurrent demyelination and remyelination is onion-bulb formation (OBF). Paraffin-embedded material is very poor at showing these structures; plastic sections are much more reliable. OBF consists of multiple axons covered by a concentric Schwann cell lamella. It is found predominantly in primary demyelination (**Figure 27.1b**). It is commonly associated with CIDP and Refsum disease, but rarely associated with CMTD (**Table 27.3**)

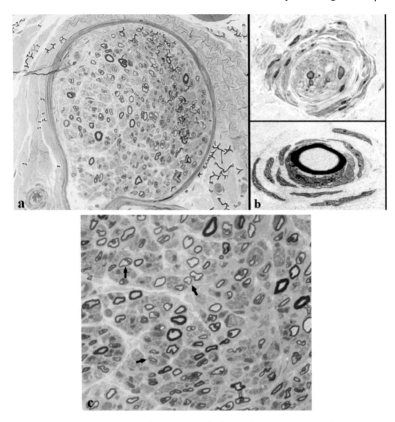

Figure 27.1 Toluidine sections of patients with demyelinating neuropathy. **(a)** Partial loss of myelination. **(b)** Onion-bulb formations as a result of demyelination-remyelination process. **(c)** Thinly myelinated fibers due to remyelination.

Table 27.2 Pathological features of demyelinating neuropathy and remyelination.

Pathology	Pathological findings
Demyelination	Complete or partial loss of myelin sheath
	Onion-bulb appearance
	Perivascular or endoneurial inflammatory infiltrate
	<u>EM</u>: Stepped paranodal demyelination, myelin loops, folded myelin, widely spaced or uncompacted myelin, tomacula
Remyelination	Thinly myelinated sheaths, onion-bulb formation

---

Table 27.3 Differential diagnosis of common pathological abnormalities affecting myelination process in peripheral nerve diseases.

Abnormality	Differential diagnosis
Onion-bulb appearance	CIDPN, Refsum disease, CMTS, toxins, Hypothyroidism, LD
Schwann cell hyperplasia	Giant axonal neuropathy
Schwann cell inclusions	Leprosy, viral, toxins, chemotherapy, glycogenosis
Lysosome inclusions	Amiodarone toxicity, glycogenosis
Extensive Reich granules	Diabetes, paraproteinemia
Widely spaced myelin	Extensive hypotonic solution, CIDP, Paraproteinemia
Uncompacted myelin	POEMS, CIDP, CMTD, lymphoma, paraproteinemia
Tomacula	Paraproteinemia, hereditary pressure sensory neuropathy

Abbreviations: CIDP: chronic inflammatory demyelinating neuropathy. CMTD: Charcot–Marie–Tooth disease. LD: leukodystrophy. POEM: polyneuropathy, organomegaly, endocrinopathy, monoclonal gammopathy, and skin changes.

One of the rare features of demyelination is abnormal myelin periodicity. The normal periodicity in fixed nerve tissue is 18 nm. Increased periodicity (>20 nm) has been observed in many demyelinating diseases of peripheral nerves (**Figure 27.2**). In uncompacted myelin (UCM), there is a space between

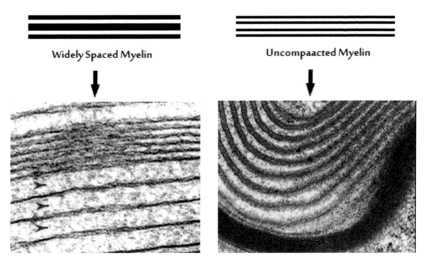

Widely Spaced Myelin

Uncompaacted Myelin

Figure 27.2 Abnormal periodicity of myelin. The diagram illustrates widely spaced myelin (WSM) formation versus uncompacted myelin (UCM) appearance.

two dense lines in which the inner and outer layers of Schwann cell cytoplasm are uncompacted. This results from disruption of remyelination. The most common demyelinating diseases associated with UCM are POEM syndrome, CIDP, and toxic myopathy.

Widely spaced myelin (WSM) is characterized by separation of interperiod lines causing increased distancing by extracellular compartment (**Figure 27.2**). The most common diseases associated with WSM are IgM-paraproteinemia and inflammatory demyelination polyneuropathy.

UCM and WSM can help in the differential diagnosis but they are not considered clear-cut features for any specific pathology.

In **Table 27.3**, we summarize the differential diagnosis of common pathological abnormalities affecting the myelination.

In summary, it is difficult to distinguish demyelinating neuropathy from axonal degeneration with secondary demyelination. Macrophage infiltration, OBF, and abnormal myelin periodicity may sometimes help. It is also difficult to distinguish the remyelination process from axonal regeneration through histopathology; however, ultrastructural examination of the tissue is important. Pathologists should inspect patient clinical history and correlate it with the pathological findings in nerve biopsy.

References

Ballin RH, Thomas PK. Electron microscope observations on demyelination and remyelination in experimental allergic neuritis. 2 Remyelination. J Neurol Sci. 1996; 8: 225–237.

Brechenmacher C, Vital C, Deminiere C, et al. Guillain-Barre syndrome: an ultrastructural study of peripheral nerve in 65 patients. Clin Neuropathol. 1987; 6: 19–24.

Jacobs JM, Scadding JW. Morphological changes in IgM paraproteinaemic neuropathy. Acta Neuropathol. 1990; 80: 77–84.

King RHM, Thomas PK. The occurrence and significance of myelin with unusually large periodicity. Acta Neuropathol. 1984; 63: 319–329.

Smith KJ, Hall SM. Peripheral demyelination and remyelination initiated by the calcium-selective ionophore ionomycin: in vivo observations. J Neurol Sci. 1988; 83: 37–53.

Vallat JM, Leboutet MJ, Jauberteau MO, et al. Widenings of the myelin lamellae in a typical Guillain-Barre syndrome. Muscle Nerve. 1994; 17: 378–380.

Vital C, Brechenmacher C, Reiffers J, et al. Uncompacted myelin lamellae in two cases of peripheral neuropathy. Acta Neuropathol. 1983; 60: 252–256.

Vital C, Gherardi R, Vital A, et al. Uncompacted myelin lamellae in polyneuropathy, organomegaly, endocrinopathy, M-protein and skin changes syndrome. Ultrastructural study of peripheral nerve biopsy from 22 patients. Acta Neuropathol. 1994; 87: 302–307.

CHAPTER 28

CELLULAR AND EXTRACELLULAR ABNORMALITIES

Recognition of intracellular and extracellular abnormalities is an important step in interpreting nerve biopsies. These abnormalities can occur in any layer of nerve fascicle. In order to identify all cellular-related structures, pathologists should start examining the paraffin sections followed by toluidine sections. The paraffin sections highlight these abnormalities morphologically better than epoxy-embedded sections. Several types of cellular and extracellular abnormalities affecting peripheral nerves are summarized in **Table 28.1** and **Table 28.2**.

Cellular abnormalities include any infiltration of the nerve fascicle or blood vessels by inflammatory cells, malignant cells, or infections. Extracellular abnormalities include any abnormal deposition of extracellular materials around or inside the nerve fascicle.

When an active inflammatory infiltrate is detected, the cell types should be identified. Perivascular cuffing with mononuclear cells is a common observation and is more readily recognized with CD45 immunostaining. They can be seen in normal nerves or in non-inflammatory neuropathies. Pathologists should be careful in interpreting these cells as they may be confused with microvasculitis. Therefore, it is better to call this kind of inflammatory infiltrate *perivascular cuffing*. CD4, CD8 and CD20 markers should also be done to rule out inflammation. The presence of neutrophils inside the blood vessel lumen is considered insignificant whereas the presence of lymphocytes within the lumen is very significant, as it raises the suspicion of vasculitic diseases.

The relationship between the inflammation and the nerve layer is important. Epineurial perivascular inflammation is usually insignificant, but it can be associated with diabetic neuropathy and leprous neuropathy. Endoneurial

Table 28.1 Cellular abnormalities in peripheral nerve diseases.

Inflammatory infiltration	Stains	Diseases
T-lymphocytes	CD4 and CD8	IDP, vasculitis
B-lymphocytes	CD20 and CD19	Lymphoma, vasculitis
T and B lymphocytes	CD4 and CD20	Vasculitis, leprosy, Lyme disease
Macrophage	CD68	AIDP, acute axonal neuropathy
Plasma cells	CD138	Lyme disease, leprosy, plasma cell diseases
Eosinophils	None	Parasitic infection, necrotizing vasculitis, HIV
Neutrophils	None	Bacterial infection, necrotizing vasculitis
Epithelioid histocytes	None	Leprosy, sarcoidosis
Granuloma	Gram stain	Leprosy, sarcoidosis, PAN
Tumor infiltration		
Malignant lymphocytes	Lymphoma markers	Lymphoma
Carcinomatous cells	CKCAM5.2, CK7, CK20	Carcinoma
Infection		
Parasites	Giemsa stain	Trypanosoma, toxoplasma, leishmania
Bacteria	Wade Fite or ZNS	Leprosy, TB, Borrelia Burgdorferi
Viruses	CMV stain	CMV, HIV, HSV, Chikungunya

Abbreviations: IDP: inflammatory demyelinating polyneuropathy. AIDP: acute inflammatory demyelinating poly-neuropathy. TB: tuberculosis. CMV: cytomegalovirus. HIV: human immunodeficiency virus. ZNS: Ziehl-Neelsen stain, PAN: polyarthritis nodosa. HSV: herpes simplex virus.

inflammation is more significant as it is commonly seen in inflammatory demyelinating polyneuropathy (IDN)

Perineurial inflammation has been reported in leprosy, sarcoidosis, cryoglobulinemia, and idiopathic perineuritis. The discrimination between the types of lymphocytic lineage is important. This will help to shorten the differential diagnosis and helps the pathologist in the interpretation.

Table 28.2 Extracellular abnormalities seen in some peripheral nerve diseases.

Extracellular abnormal deposition	Location	Stain	Disease
Calcification	Perineurium	Von-Kossa	Diabetes, leprosy, amiodarone
Amyloid fibrils	Endoneurium and perivascular	Congo red	Amyloidosis
Glycogen	Endoneurium	PAS	Glycogenosis, cryoglobulinemia
Myxoid changes	Subperineurium	None	Hypothyroidism, POEMS

Abbreviations: PAS: periodic acid-Schiff. POEMS: polyneuropathy, organomegaly, endocrinopathy, monoclonal gammopathy, and skin changes.

Immunohistochemistry (IHC) is a required tool to differentiate between cellular types. Predominant T-lymphocytes are associated with IDN and some types of vasculitis. B-lymphocytic lineage is commonly seen in lymphoma particularly when fascicular infiltration is detected. Mixed types of T and B-lymphocytes can also be seen in IDN; however, leprosy and Lyme disease should be ruled out.

Endoneurial or epineurial macrophages are a common finding in acute axonal degeneration or acute inflammatory demyelinating polyneuropathy (AIDN). Other cellular inflammatory cells are summarized in **Table 28.1**.

Infectious neuropathy due to bacterial, viral, or parasitic infections is rare in clinical practice. The most common infection affecting the nerve is *leprous neuropathy*. It is a mycobacterial infection, common in the underdeveloped world, and characterized by acid-fast and gram-positive bacilli, 1–8 μm in length. Neuronal involvement always occurs early and invariable. It has a predilection for Schwann cells. Most patients are classified into two spectrums: tuberculoid or lepromatous. Unfortunately, there is no sensitive serological test to detect leprosy. Consequently, the diagnosis is always established on clinical grounds. Most leprosy patients develop IgM against PGL-1 (phenolic glycolipid) antibody. Patients clinically present with symmetrical sensory neuropathy commonly affecting the distal part of limbs. Skin changes are very common in lepromatous neuropathy and facial involvement occurs in severe cases. Damage to peripheral nerves occurs before and after treatment and can result in long-term disability. Because leprosy directly affects peripheral nerves without skin manifestations, the diagnosis with nerve biopsy is recommended.

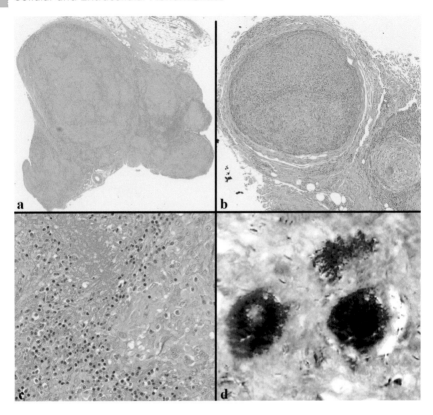

Figure 28.1 Histological sections from a 28-year-old patient with leprous neuropathy. **(a–c)** H&E sections with different magnifications show multiple necrotizing endoneurial granulomas. **(d)** Section with Fite stain shows foamy cells and scattered mycobacterial bacilli. ×40.

Histologically, it is characterized by perineuritis with endoneurial necrotizing granulomas. The presence of multibacillary in nerves and paucibacillary in skin is a common finding. Macrophages and Schwann cells are filled with foamy-lepra cells. In the perineurium, foamy macrophages infiltrate to form individual layers of fibroblasts, perineurial cells, and collagens producing an "onion skinning" of the nerve fascicles (**Figure 28.1a–c**). The Fite Faraco technique is the oldest method used to detect mycobacterium leprae in tissue specimens (**Figure 28.1d**). Microvasculitis and perineurial calcifications are also observed in leprosy. The disease may progress to cause severe axonal degeneration affecting both myelinated and unmyelinated fibers. Regenerating clusters may be found. In electron microscopy (EM), rod-shaped electron-dense structures surrounded by clear halos are seen. Large numbers of macrophages with foamy appearance, which contain bacilli, may be present.

Neuropathy due to viral infection causes acute inflammatory demyelinating neuropathy (AIDN)-like syndrome. Although it is difficult to identify viral inclusions within the nerve fascicles, lymphocytic infiltration with axonal pathology can be seen. Demyelinating neuropathy has also been observed in many cases. The best method for diagnosis is serological blood test. Latent virus is not visible by EM, but the viral genome can usually be demonstrated with a mild lymphocytic infiltrate.

Extracellular abnormalities include any abnormal deposition of extracellular materials in nerve fascicle (**Table 28.2**). The most common non-specific extracellular deposition in the nerve tissue is perineurial calcification. It is often not detected in nerve biopsy because tissue preparation causes its removal. Extensive microcalcifications may be seen in diabetic neuropathy, leprosy, or amiodarone toxicity. Focal traumatic injury might sometimes be accompanied by microcalcifications. Other extracellular materials are summarized in **Table 28.2** and will be discussed in detail in *Chapter 30.*

References

Boddingius J. Ultrastructural changes in blood vessels of peripheral nerves in leprosy neuropathy. II. Borderline, borderline –lepromatous, and lepromatous leprosy patients. Acta Neuropathol. 1977; 40: 21–39.

Finlayson MH, Bilbao JM, Lough JO. The pathogenesis of the neuropathy in dimorphous leprosy: electron microscopic and cytochemical studies. J Neuropathol Exp Neurol. 1974; 33: 446–455.

Jacobs JM, Shetty VP, Antia NH. A morphological study of nerve biopsies from cases of multibacillary leprosy given multidrug therapy. Acta Neuropathol. 1993; 85: 533–541.

Paetau A, Haltia M. Calcification of the perineurium. A case report. Acta Neuropathol. 1985; 36: 185–191.

Pearson JMH, Weddell AGM. Perineurial changes in leprosy. Lepr Rev. 1975; 46: 51–67.

Schroder JM. Proliferation of epineurial capillaries and smooth muscle cells in angiopathic peripheral neuropathy. Acta Neuropathol. 1986; 72: 29–37.

Vallat JM, Leboutet MJ, Henry P, et al. Endoneurial proliferation of perineurial cells in leprosy. Acta Neuropathol. 1971; 81: 336–338.

Vital C, Heraud A, Vital A, et al. Acute mononeuropathy with angiotropic lymphoma. Acta Neuropathol. 1989; 78: 105–107.

CHAPTER 29

INFLAMMATORY DEMYELINATION

Contents

Inflammatory demyelinating neuropathy (IDN) is a rare neurological disease in clinical practice, but it is one of the most common forms of peripheral neuropathy. It is classified as an acquired immune-mediated inflammatory disease of undetermined etiology, in which the myelin sheath surrounding the axons is attacked by the immune system. It is presumed to occur because of antibody-mediated reaction along with infiltration of the endoneurium and blood vessels with T-cell lymphocytes and macrophages. The consequence is a segmental demyelination.

The disease is clinically manifested with slowly progressive sensory and motor deficits in the upper or lower limbs. The hallmark sign for the diagnosis is evidence of demyelination seen in electrodiagnostic studies. The nerve biopsy is used as a confirmatory method for the diagnosis, in which inflammatory demyelination is the hallmark feature.

IDN is subclassified into two types:

1. Acute inflammatory demyelinating neuropathy (AIDN)
2. Chronic inflammatory demyelinating neuropathy (CIDN)

29.1 Acute Inflammatory Demyelinating Neuropathy (AIDN)—Guillain–Barré Syndrome (GBS)

AIDN, or GBS, is a rare neurological disease that affects two cases per 100,000 throughout the world. It is a rapidly progressive disease characterized by the presence of demyelination and inflammation. Despite the presence of different variants, most cases are typical and the diagnosis can be established clinically. However, it is difficult to distinguish AIDN from other immune-mediated inflammatory neuropathies, so a nerve biopsy may be required.

The exact cause of GBS is unknown. Two-thirds of patients report symptoms after viral infection or post-vaccination in the 6 weeks preceding. These include cytomegalovirus, Epstein-Barr virus, HIV, and Zika virus.

Patients clinically present with acute-onset and progressive sensory and motor deficits over a month with complete absence of limb reflexes. The deficits are usually symmetrical and ascending in fashion. It may progress to involve facial nerve and respiratory muscles, which later requires dependent ventilation. AIDN cases progressing beyond 8 weeks should be categorized as chronic inflammatory demyelinating neuropathy (CIDN).

Cerebrospinal fluid (CSF) shows elevated levels of proteins with normal cell counts. Nerve conduction test (NCT) may show subtle changes of demyelinating pattern. Although the axons are always preserved, two variants of GBS are associated with axonal degeneration: acute motor axonal neuropathy (AMAN) and acute motor and sensory axonal neuropathy (AMSAN). Sensory action potential is usually normal in AMAN compared to AMSAN, which has absent sensory action potential.

Serological tests for patients with IDN may help in the diagnosis. In patients with GBS, circulating antiganglioside antibodies are found in high concentration more than in non-inflammatory neuropathies. AMAN and AMSAN are associated with serum IgG binding to GM1, GD1a, and GalNAc-GD1a gangliosides. Although antibodies against gangliosides (GM1, GM2, basal lamina components, and several myelin proteins) have been identified in some cases, no characteristic pattern of anti-ganglioside antibodies has been established in AIDN.

AMAN/AMSAN may confuse the clinician or pathologist with the diagnosis of axonal neuropathy with secondary demyelination. There are some clinical differences between classical AIDN and AMAN. For example, areflexia is a major criterion required to make a diagnosis of GBS, but patients with AMAN usually have normal or exaggerated reflexes. Pathologically, axonal involvement in demyelinating neuropathy turns the diagnosis toward AMAN or AMSAN.

Nerve biopsy in GBS is not always recommended because the syndrome is easily diagnosed on clinical grounds. Biopsy is suggested when the clinical presentations are atypical or vasculitic neuropathy is in the differential. The histopathological hallmark of AIDN is evidence of active demyelination with inflammation; the latter mainly consists of mononuclear inflammatory cells infiltrate and CD4+ T-lymphocytes. The inflammation can be seen perivascular or endoneurial. Some cases may show subperineurial macrophages. Myelin debris-filled macrophages are seen in the endoneurium and usually are of perivascular distribution. The axons are always preserved. Axonal loss is considered as "bystander effect" due to endoneurial cytokine accumulation. The severity of these changes depends on the duration of the disease. Some cases show selective involvement of large myelinated fibers. Loss of unmyelinated fibers and remyelination can also be seen in AIDN.

Axonal GBS (AMAN or AMSAN) is difficult to differentiate from classical GBS or axonal degeneration with secondary demyelination. We can say lack of inflammation, minimal demyelination, and extensive axonal degeneration are more common in axonal GBS than classical GBS. Unfortunately, there is no microscopic evidence to clearly distinguish these two entities. Pathologists should make comments in the diagnostic report to explain the findings in correlation with the clinical history of the patient.

29.2 Chronic Inflammatory Demyelinating Neuropathy (CIDN)

This has recently been called *chronic inflammatory demyelinating polyradiculoneuropathy* (CIDPN). Basically, it is the chronic type of inactive GBS. CIDPN is a remitting and relapsing disease with persistent evolution over many months. It is characterized by sensory and motor deficits associated with reduced reflexes. Motor symptoms tend to be more predominant than the sensory symptoms and may affect both proximal and distal limbs. CSF protein is elevated, and the cell count differential is usually normal. NCT shows predominant demyelinating patterns with variable axonal involvement. Circulating paraproteins are seen in 30% of patients. Antibody to contactin-associated protein-1 (CASPR-1) or anti-beta-tubulin antibody has been observed in high titration in cases of CIDP and CIDP-remission cases, respectively.

Several variants of CIDP have been covered in the literature. Typical CIDP is the most predominant classical subtype. Chronic immune sensory type and Lewis–Sumner syndrome are pure sensory types associated with asymmetrical distribution and predominant upper limb involvement. The difference between AIDN and CIDP is in the onset and progression. AIDP has a very rapid and aggressive course compared to CIDP. The distinction between recurrent GBS and relapsing CIDP is also difficult.

Histologically, the essential diagnostic features of CIDP in nerve biopsy are segmental demyelination, excessive remyelination, with or without onion-bulb formations (OBFs) (**Figure 29.1**). Inflammation is uncommon and occurs in 0%–50% of cases. Macrophages containing myelin debris, T-cell lymphocytes, and up-regulation of major histocompatibility complex (MHC) class II expression, lack of B-cell infiltration, subperineurial and endoneurial edema are other associated histopathological features. Pro-inflammatory cytokine expression invariably shows interleukin-1 in perivascular and endoneurial ramified cells.

Although myelinated axon numbers can be normal even if the disease is in its active status, mixed axonal degeneration-demyelination occurs in many CIDP cases. Presence of OBFs in the nerve section supports the demyelinating nature of the disease and indicates the recurrent demyelination-remyelination process. The demyelinating nature of the process may be hard to appreciate if only a few thinly myelinated or naked axons are seen (**Figure 29.1c**).

Because histological features of CIDN are difficult to differentiate from axonal degeneration with regeneration, clinical correlation is recommended. Evidence of post-treatment response also confirms the diagnosis.

Ultrastructural examination of EM sections usually shows non-specific findings. Macrophages containing myelin debris, scattered OBFs, and thinly myelinated fibers may be present.

Distinguishing CIDP from other inflammatory neuropathies is also difficult histologically. Some of the common differential diagnoses are vasculitic neuropathy (VN) and Charcot–Marie–Tooth syndrome (CMTS). CIDP and VN may both involve myelinated axons and coexist with inflammation. However, the axonal involvement in VN is more pronounced (**Table 29.2**). There is no abnormal myelin periodicity seen in VN. In CMTS, endoneurial lymphocytic perivascular cuffs and macrophage-mediated myelin stripping are not seen, compared to CIDP. Signs of active demyelination are not present in CMTS. CIDP should also be distinguished from familial hypertrophic neuropathy; the latter is characterized by extensive OBFs with lack of inflammation.**Table 29.1** summarizes the clinicopathological features of AIDP and CIDN. **Table 29.2** outlines how to differentiate between IDN and VN.

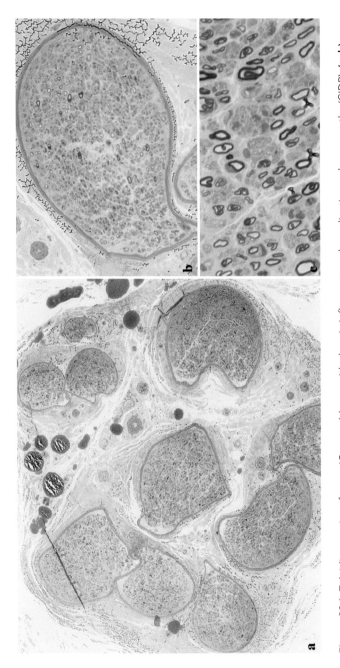

Figure 29.1 Toluidine sections from a 65-year-old man with chronic inflammatory demyelinating polyneuropathy (CIDP). **(a, b)** Lower-magnification sections show diffuse demyelination with evidence of remyelination. **(c)** Section of high magnification shows evidence of extensive remyelination.

Table 29.1 The clinicopathological features differentiating AIDN, CIDP, and axonal degeneration with secondary demyelination.

	AIDN or GBS	CIDN or CIDP	Axonal degeneration
Onset	Days to weeks	>8 weeks	Variable
Antibodies	Antiganglioside antibodies	Not detected; CASPR1	Not detected
Progression	Rapid	Remitting-relapsing	Variable
Demyelination	Active	Chronic	Active to chronic
Inflammation	Common >50%	Rare <50%	No
Remyelination	Rare	Extensive	No
Regeneration	No	No	Yes
Axonal involvement	Rare (only in AMAN)	Common	Predominant
Myelin-filled macrophages	Present	Rare	Rare
Unmyelinated fibers	Common	Variable	Rare
Onion-bulb formations	Rare	Common	No

Abbreviations: AIDN: acute inflammatory demyelinating neuropathy. GBS: Guillain–Barre syndrome. CIDN: chronic inflammatory demyelinating neuropathy or polyneuropathy. CASPR-1: contactin associated-protein 1. AMAN: acute motor axonal neuropathy.

Table 29.2 Histological differentiation between inflammatory demyelinating neuropathy (IDN) and vasculitic neuropathy (VN).

Inflammatory demyelinating neuropathy	Vasculitic neuropathy
Epineurial or perivascular lymphocytic inflammation	Perivascular mixed lymphocytic inflammation
Primary demyelination	Secondary demyelination
Rare axonal degeneration or axonal sparing	Marked axonal degeneration
Macrophage-containing myelin debris	Granuloma can be present
No evidence of fibrinoid necrosis	Fibrinoid necrosis can be present
Widely spaced myelin or uncompacted myelin	No abnormal myelin periodicity

References

Arstila AU, Riekkinen PJ, Rinne UK, et al. Guillain-Barre syndrome. Neurochemical and ultrastructural study. Eur Neurol. 1971; 5: 257–269.

Austin JH. Observations on the syndrome of hypertrophic neuritis (the hypertrophic interstitial radiculoneuropathies). Medicine. 1956; 35: 187–237

Barohn RJ, Kissel JT, Warmolts JR, et al. Chronic inflammatory demyelinating polyradiculoneuropathy. Clinical characteristics, course, and recommendations for diagnostic criteria. Arch Neurol. 1989; 46: 878–884.

Berciano J, Coria F, Monton F, et al. Axonal form of Guillain-Barre syndrome: evidence for macrophage mediated demyelination. Muscle Nerve. 1993; 16: 744–751.

Brechenmacher C, Vital C, Deminiere C, et al. Guillain–Barre syndrome: an ultrastructural study of peripheral nerve in 65 patients. Clin Neuropathol. 1987; 6: 19–24.

Connolly AM, Pestronk A, Trotter JL, et al. High-titer selective serum anti-beta-tubulin antibodies in chronic inflammatory demyelinating polyneuropathy. Neurology. 1983; 43: 557–562.

Dyck PJ, Lais AC, Ohta M, et al. Chronic inflammatory polyradiculoneuropathy. Mayo Clin Proc. 1975; 50: 621–637.

Feasby TE, Hahn AF, Brown WF, et al. Severe axonal degeneration in acute Guillain-Barre syndrome: evidence of two different mechanisms. J Neurol Sci. 1993; 116: 185–192.

Gorson KC, Katz J. Chronic inflammatory demyelinating polyneuropathy. Neurol Clin. 2013; 31: 511–532.

Griffin JW, Stoll G, Li CY, et al. Macrophage responses in inflammatory demyelinating neuropathies. Ann Neurol. 1990; S64–S68.

Ho TW, Willison HJ, Nachamkin I, et al. Anti-GD1a antibody is associated with axonal but not demyelinating forms of Guillain-Barre syndrome. Ann Neurol. 1999; 45: 168–173.

Julien J, Vital C, Lagueny A, et al. Chronic relapsing idiopathic polyneuropathy with primary axonal lesions. J Neurol Neurosurg Psychiatry. 1989; 52: 871–875.

Kornberg AJ, Pestronk K. The clinical and diagnostic role of anti–GM1 antibody testing. Muscle Nerve. 1994; 17: 100–104.

Krendel DA, Parks HP, Anthony DC, et al. Sural nerve biopsy in chronic inflammatory demyelinating polyradiculoneuropathy. Muscle Nerve. 1989; 12: 257–264.

Madrid RE, Wisniewski HM. Axonal degeneration in demyelinating disorders. J Neurocytol. 1977; 6: 103–117.

Rizzuto N, Morbin M, Cavallaro T, et al. Focal lesions area feature of chronic inflammatory demyelinating polyneuropathy. Acta Neuropathologica. 1998; 96(6): 603–609.

Vriesendorp FJ, Mishu B, Blaser MJ, et al. Serum antibodies to GM1, GD1b, peripheral nerve myelin, and campylobacter jejuni in patients with Guillain–Barre syndrome and controls: correlation and prognosis. Ann Neurol. 1993; 34: 130–135.

CHAPTER 30

OTHER COMMON PERIPHERAL NEUROPATHIES

Several groups of peripheral nerve diseases are rarely seen in clinical practice. Most of them are diagnosed clinically and may not require nerve biopsy. The biopsy should be performed to confirm the diagnosis or to detect disease remission status. Using the approach in *Chapter 25* with additional knowledge from this chapter will improve the diagnostic abilities. In this chapter, we summarize some common conditions of rare peripheral nerve disorders seen in the clinical practice. We describe their causes, clinical features, and pathological findings.

Vasculitis neuropathy (VN) is an inflammatory vasculitis of peripheral nerves. It can occur as an isolated process or can be associated with other systemic diseases (**Table 30.1**). It is characterized histologically with perivascular inflammation mainly seen in the endoneurium and perineurium and associated with axonal degeneration. The most common clinical presentation of VN is mononeuritis multiplex and symmetrical distal polyneuropathies. The patients always have axonal degeneration patterns in nerve conduction tests (NCTs). A coexisting demyelinating pattern may be seen. Eosinophilia and rheumatological manifestations are the red flags in the diagnosis of VN. The clinician should exclude ANCA-associated vasculitis and connective tissue diseases such as systemic lupus erythematosus (SLE) and rheumatoid arthritis (RA).

The sensitivity of nerve biopsy in cases suspected to have vasculitis is unknown. Hellmman et al. (1988) biopsied 35 patients with mononeuritis multiplex and variable systemic and rheumatological diseases. Three patients, with clinically proven polyarteritis nodosa (PAN), showed definitive vasculitis on nerve biopsy.

Histologically, the biopsy shows typical chronic axonal degeneration with perivascular CD4+ lymphocytic inflammation mainly seen in the perineurium. Endoneurial inflammation is uncommon and may occasionally be called "hypersensitivity vasculitis." Therefore, VN should be differentiated from CIDPN where endoneurial inflammation can be seen. (See *Chapter 29, Table 29.2*.) If there is no microscopic evidence of necrotic vasculopathy, it is not possible to call it vasculitis. Fibrinoid necrosis, thrombosis, and focal hemorrhages are the standard features for necrotizing vasculitis (**Figure 30.1**). These features are commonly seen in giant cell arteritis and some ANCA-associated vasculopathies. Muscle biopsy is also encouraged for patients suspected to have VN.

Large myelinated axons are usually affected, and the disease may show regenerating clusters in recovery period. Demyelination can occur in VN, based on the severity of the axonal degeneration. Remote VN is characterized histological by narrowing of blood vessel lumen, luminal thrombosis, intimal hyperplasia, sclerosis, old hemorrhage, and focal microcalcifications.

In conclusion, VN can be diagnosed through nerve biopsy but is very difficult to differentiate it from other inflammatory neuropathies. Good clinical history and reliable inspection of nerve tissue would assist the pathologist in the diagnosis.

Paraproteinemic neuropathy is characterized by the presence of circulating monoclonal immunoglobulins and peripheral neuropathy. It may occur as an idiopathic form or be associated with other systemic diseases. **Table 30.1** summarizes the systemic diseases associated with paraproteinemia. Monoclonal gammopathy of unknown significance (MCGUS) due to clonal expansion of B-cell lineage or multiple myeloma due to plasma cell expansion are the most common forms associated with this paraproteinemic neuropathy. MCGUS is clinically diagnosed when monoclonal protein is less than 30 g/L with normal kidney and blood functions. The most common protein type is IgG and IgM.

Patients usually present with slowly progressive and symmetrical distal sensorimotor neuropathy with variable nerve distributions (painful mononeuritis multiplex-like picture). In nerve biopsy, the histological features are usually non-specific. There is a variable degree of segmental demyelination and axonal degeneration. Endoneurial lymphocytic inflammation with plasmacytoid infiltrate is common. Three pathological features characterize paraproteinemic neuropathy from other types of neuropathies: perineurial vacuolation, subperineurial amorphous material (+ for PAS and IgM), and widely spaced myelin in ultrastructural sections (**Figure 30.2**). Because paraproteinemia is uncommonly seen in clinical practice, the clinician rarely asks for nerve biopsy. The biopsy may only be done to evaluate the disease progression when treatment does not show efficient results.

Cryoglobulinemic neuropathy is one of the causes of neuropathy in neurological practice. The most common subtype is IgM. Mixed

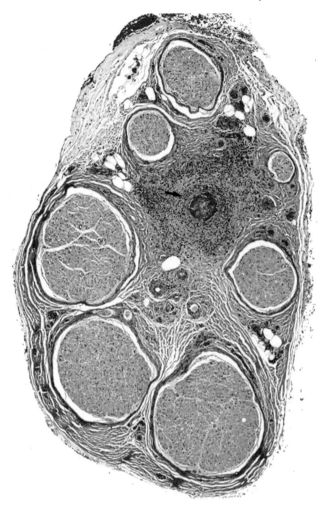

Figure 30.1 H&E section of multiple nerves from a patient with vasculitic neuropathy. There is a focal area of perivascular necrotizing inflammation with fibrinoid necrosis (*black arrow*). ×5. Reprinted by permission from Springer Nature, Biopsy diagnosis of Peripheral Neuropathy, by Juan M. Bilbao and Robert E. Schmidt, 2nd Ed Copyright, 2015.

cryoglobulinemia is associated with hepatitis C virus infection. Chronic patients present with distal sensorimotor neuropathy and mononeuritis-like syndrome. The most common remarkable finding in nerve biopsy is marked perineuritis. The inflammation may infiltrate to involve the endoneurium.

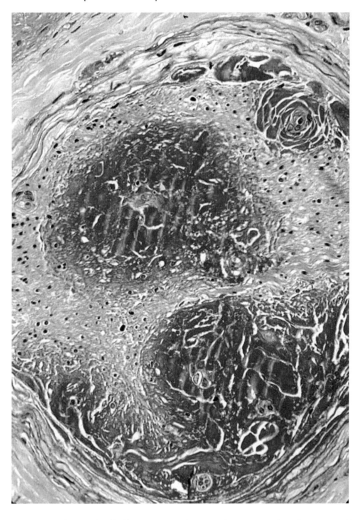

Figure 30.2 Periodic acid-Schiff (PAS) stain shows subperineurial and perivascular deposition of amorphous materials that indicates paraproteinemic neuropathy. Reprinted by permission from Springer Nature, Biopsy diagnosis of Peripheral Neuropathy, by Juan M. Bilbao and Robert E. Schmidt, 2nd Ed Copyright, 2015.

Axonal degeneration with regeneration and relative sparing of unmyelinated fibers are usually seen.

Amyloid neuropathy is defined as widespread amyloidosis that affects multiple nerves. It could be familial such as familial amyloid polyneuropathy (FAP) or non-familial (primary or secondary subtypes). FAP is associated with apolipoprotein Ig-light chain. It usually occurs as an isolated neuropathy. Primary amyloidosis occurs in 50% of cases and is associated with paraprotein deposition and underlying plasma cell diseases such as multiple myeloma. The clinical diagnosis is always established before the biopsy. Patients may present with painful symmetrical distal sensorimotor neuropathy associated with muscle weakness. Findings of monoclonal free-light chain or plasma cells in bone marrow biopsy and urinary test are suggestive for primary amyloidosis. Secondary amyloidosis is the rarest causative variant of amyloid neuropathy because it is not always present with peripheral neuropathy. Secondary amyloidosis is commonly associated with systemic chronic inflammatory diseases.

Nerve biopsy for patients with probable amyloidosis is sensitive for the diagnosis. Muscle biopsy is considered much more sensitive and reliable. The most common specific histological finding is the presence of amyloid deposits in the epineurium, intraperineurium, subperineurium, and endoneurium, and within the hyalinized blood vessels (**Figure 30.3**). These deposits are described as foci of amorphous masses or fine fibrils that are visualized as red on Congo red stain or light-green birefringence under polarized microscope. This morphology may be diluted with formalin-fixed paraffin-embedded tissue sections. Thioflavin T or S can be used as an alternative for Congo red if amyloid was not detected in highly suspected cases. Axonal degeneration with regeneration or segmental degeneration may be seen in most cases. The

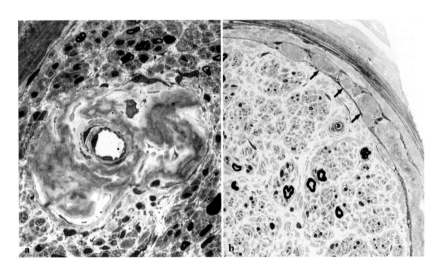

Figure 30.3 Toluidine section from a peripheral nerve of a patient with amyloid neuropathy. **(a)** Perivascular amyloid deposition. **(b)** Small clumps of subperineurial amyloid (*black arrow*). ×40. Reprinted by permission from Springer Nature, Biopsy diagnosis of Peripheral Neuropathy, by Juan M. Bilbao and Robert E. Schmidt, 2nd Ed Copyright, 2015.

amyloid fibrils (8–13 nm) are best seen ultrastructurally using EM sections (*Figure 12.1i, Chapter 12*).

Paraneoplastic neuropathy occurs when neurological symptoms develop Within 1-5 years prior to cancer diagnosis. It also includes patients with paraneoplastic manifestations during their cancer period. The cancers most associated with neuropathy are small-cell carcinoma of the lung, hematological malignancies, and breast carcinoma. Antibodies to Hu and Yo are rarely identified. Patients typically present with subacute sensory neuropathy and autonomic dysfunction.

The hallmark histological sign in nerve biopsy is vasculitic neuropathy (VN). When lymphoma is suspected, infiltrated neoplastic lymphocytes are seen throughout the endoneurium (**Figure 30.4**). Intravascular lymphocytes may also be seen in the lumen of epineurial microvessels. CD8, CD20, and CD10 should be performed to classify the lymphomas. For carcinomas, CK7, CK20, and TTF-1 immunomarkers should be investigated to segregate the types of

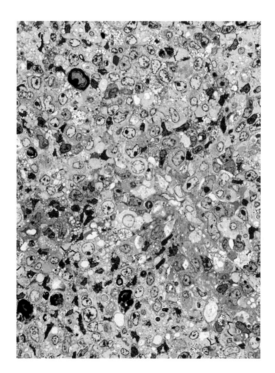

Figure 30.4 Toluidine section from a peripheral nerve of a patient with lymphomatous neuropathy. There is a diffuse neoplastic lymphocyte in the endoneurium. Reprinted by permission from Springer Nature, Biopsy diagnosis of Peripheral Neuropathy, by Juan M. Bilbao and Robert E. Schmidt, 2nd Ed Copyright, 2015.

malignancy. Paraneoplastic neuropathy can progress to affect the muscle tissue causing neuromyopathy or autoimmune necrotizing myopathy (see *Chapter 14*).

Diabetic neuropathy (DN) is the most common form of acquired systemic neuropathy in neuromuscular practice. There are two clinical spectrums of DN: (1) painful symmetrical distal sensorimotor neuropathy, and (2) painless symmetrical proximal amyotrophy (diabetic polyradiculopathy). The latter is associated with cranial nerve palsies or autonomic dysfunction. Performing nerve biopsy in diabetic patients with neuropathic features is required when the disease progresses into muscle wasting and severe loss of sensation.

The hallmark histopathological feature in nerve biopsy is chronic axonal degeneration with minimal regenerations. Both large and small myelinated fibers are depleted. In late stage, segmental demyelination may occur. Thickness and hyalinization of endoneurial microvessels are common microscopic features of DN (**Figure 30.5**). In conclusion, DN should be suspected in any

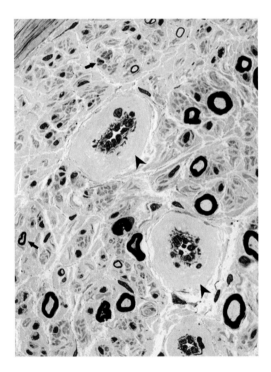

Figure 30.5 Toluidine nerve section from a patient with diabetic neuropathy. There is axonal degeneration with regeneration (*black arrow*). Marked thickenings of blood vessel walls are well-visualized (*arrowhead*). Reprinted by permission from Springer Nature, Biopsy diagnosis of Peripheral Neuropathy, by Juan M. Bilbao and Robert E. Schmidt, 2nd Ed Copyright, 2015.

case with chronic diabetes presenting neuropathy. The diagnosis is established clinically but the nerve biopsy may be used as a confirmatory tool.

Alcoholic neuropathy is common in western countries. These patients present with painful symmetrical and distal sensorimotor neuropathy with complete absence of reflexes. History of heavy alcohol drinking is the only way to relate the clinical presentation with pathological findings. The main histological feature is axonal degeneration with regeneration. There is no specific morphological sign associated with alcoholic neuropathy. In very rare cases, segmental demyelination coexists. The diagnosis of alcoholic neuropathy is very difficult through nerve biopsy. It may be expected when the alcoholic patient presents only with neuropathy, free from other abnormal systemic conditions.

Abnormal deposition of exogenous substances, including medications, metals, and biological toxins, in peripheral nerves is called *toxic neuropathy.* This deposition occurs when the toxin is taken either in a suicidal dose or in high therapeutic doses for a long duration. The clinical presentation is variable and dependent on the dose and the duration. The main clinical features are sensory rather than motor neuropathy (**Table 30.1**). Pathologists should read carefully the clinical history when toxic neuropathy is suspected. Clinicians should provide complete patient medications lists, to include doses and durations. Nerve biopsy is always inconclusive in patients with toxic neuropathy. Nevertheless, some cases, such as lead poisoning, require biopsy for confirmation or exclusion.

The main histological sign of toxic neuropathy is axonal degeneration. Selective loss of large myelinated fibers is seen. Lysosomal inclusions of Schwann cells, perineurial cells, and endothelial cells were observed in many cases with amiodaron toxicity.

In conclusion, the diagnosis of toxic neuropathy by nerve biopsy is challenging and requires multidisciplinary team collaboration. Clinical history is very important in the diagnosis.

Charcot–Marie–Tooth disease (CMTD) is also called hereditary sensory and motor neuropathy. It encompasses heterogeneous groups of inherited demyelinating polyneuropathies with different clinical phenotypes and genetic mutations. It can be inherited as autosomal dominant or autosomal recessive, based on the underlying variant. The clinical spectrums vary in their onset and their associated genetic mutations (**Table 30.1**). We cannot include all variants here, as their histopathological features cannot be distinguished by light microcopy.

Genetic analysis is the best method for diagnosis.

Generally, patients present with symmetrical distal sensorimotor neuropathy with muscle weakness, hammer toes, and pes cavus. Skeletal abnormalities may be present. The disease affects children and slowly progress to adulthood. Hypertrophic nerve is a common finding in clinical examination and gross diagnosis of biopsied nerve. Histologically, the predominant feature is non-inflammatory demyelinating neuropathy with minimal remyelination. Unmyelinated fibers are slightly reduced in number with autosomal dominant adult cases. The pathognomonic feature of CMTD is the presence of extensive onion-bulb formations microscopically (**Figure 30.6**) and uncompacted myelin ultrastructurally. CMT-2 is the only subtype that shows predominant axonal degeneration and atrophy.

Giant axonal neuropathy (GAN) is a rare autosomal inherited disease. It occurs due to GAN gene mutation on chromosome 16q23 that encodes gigaxonin. The patient typically presents during childhood with kinky hair,

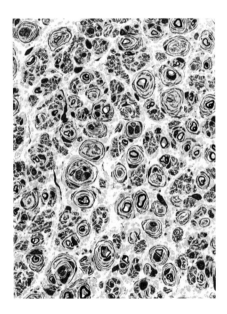

Figure 30.6 Toluidine section from a patient with Charcot–Marie–Tooth disease (CMTD) shows extensive onion-bulb formations. Reprinted by permission from Springer Nature, Biopsy diagnosis of Peripheral Neuropathy, by Juan M. Bilbao and Robert E. Schmidt, 2nd Ed Copyright, 2015.

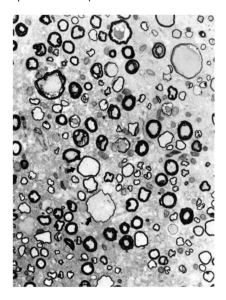

Figure 30.7 Toluidine section from a patient with giant axonal neuropathy (GAN) shows abnormally distended giant axons (*black arrow*). Reprinted by permission from Springer Nature, Biopsy diagnosis of Peripheral Neuropathy, by Juan M. Bilbao and Robert E. Schmidt, 2nd Ed Copyright, 2015.

peripheral neuropathy, white matter changes in the brain, and skeletal abnormalities. GAN does not require nerve biopsy. The diagnosis is always established through clinical ground. The presence of filamentous accumulation in the skin is enough for the diagnosis.

Nerve biopsy shows abnormal scattered distended axons that are not surrounded with myelin sheath (**Figure 30.7**). Regeneration and demyelination may be accompanied. Ultrastructurally, it shows reduplicated basal laminae and filamentous collection in the sub-axolemmal area.

In conclusion, CMTD and GAN are rare hereditary clinical spectrums of peripheral neuropathies, best diagnosed clinically. The nerve biopsy may not add actual value to the diagnosis but it may be used to evaluate the disease progression or to exclude other types of neuropathies in the differential diagnosis.

Table 30.1 Other common peripheral neuropathies.

Neuropathic disease	Causes	Clinical features	Microscopic features
Vasculitic neuropathy (VN)	Isolated vasculitis Cryoglobulinemia Rheumatological (PAN-WG-SLE-SD) Infection (Lyme disease, leprosy, HIV) Sarcoidosis Paraneoplastic (leukemia or lymphoma)	• Always adult-onset • Slowly progressive • Mononeuritis multiplex • Symmetrical distal polyneuropathy • Sensory ataxia • Other systemic features	1. Perivascular inflammation in perineurium > endoneurium 2. Chronic axonal degeneration with regeneration 3. Minimal axonal regeneration 4. Fibrinoid necrosis of microvessels (in PAN and WG) 5. Destruction of arterial muscular media and IEL 6. Old vasculitis: sclerosis, calcification, and proliferation
Paraneoplastic neuropathy	Small-cell carcinoma of lungs Breast cancer Hematological malignancies (lymphoma) **Associated with anti Hu/Yo antibodies	• Subacute sensory neuropathy • Motor neuropathy (rare) • Sensory ataxia • Autonomic dysfunction	1. Vasculitic neuropathy features 2. Axonal degeneration 3. Malignant cells (+ CK7 or TTF1 or CD3/CD20+) 4. Chronic lymphocytic infiltrate (CD8+ T-cells)

(Continued)

Table 30.1 Other common peripheral neuropathies. *(Continued)*

Neuropathic disease	Causes	Clinical features	Microscopic features
Diabetic neuropathy (DN)	Thesis-related factors: • Oxidative stress • Mitochondrial dysfunction • Insulin resistance • Axonal transport defect	• Adult-onset • Symmetrical distal sensorimotor neuropathy • Asymmetrical neuropathy (amyotrophy) • Sensory ataxia • Autonomic dysfunction	1. Axonal degeneration with regeneration 2. Hyalinization of endoneurial microvessels 3. Segmental demyelination (rare) 4. Perivascular epineuritis (in amyotrophy type) 5. Perineurial calcium inclusions 6. Extensive Reich granules 7. Duplicated basal layer of vessels in EM
Hereditary Motor Sensory Neuropathy (CMTD)	Different subtypes. The commonest: CMT-1: ADD; PMP22 duplication on Ch.17 CMT-2: ADD; MFN2 mutation on Ch. 1p36 CMT-3: ADD; Dejerine-Sottas disease CMT-4: ARD; GDAP-1 gene mutation	• Child or adult onset • Symmetrical distal sensorimotor neuropathy • Complete absence of reflexes • Pes cavus or hammer toe • Distal leg atrophy	1. Segmental demyelination with remyelination (Type I,3,4) 2. Extensive OBFs 3. Endoneurial edema 4. Axonal degeneration with regeneration (Type 2) 5. Uncompacted myelin in EM

(Continued)

Table 30.1 Other common peripheral neuropathies. *(Continued)*

Neuropathic disease	Causes	Clinical features	Microscopic features
Paraproteinemic Neuropathy	Idiopathic 10%. MCGUS Multiple myeloma Waldenstorm macroglobulinemia Lymphoproliferative diseases Cryoglobulinemia	• Adult onset • Slowly progressive • Symmetrical sensorimotor distal neuropathy • Mononeuritis multiplex-like features • Other systemic features	1. Segmental demyelination with remyelination 2. Rare axonal degeneration 3. Perivascular inflammation in endoneurium > perineurium 4. Plasmocytic infiltrate 5. Perineurial vacuolation 6. Subperineurial Ig deposition (PAS+ and IgM+) 7. OBF and widely spaced myelin
Cryoglobulinemic Neuropathy	Idiopathic. IgM > IgG Mixed type associated with Hepatitis C	• Adult onset • Slowly progressive • Symmetrical sensorimotor distal neuropathy • Mononeuritis multiplex-like features • Other systemic features	1. Axonal degeneration with regeneration 2. Perivascular inflammation in perineurium > endoneurium 3. Severe perineuritis 4. Endoneurial Ig deposition (PAS+ and IgM+) 5. Rare OBF
Alcoholic neuropathy	Direct toxic effect on the peripheral nerve or indirectly due to thiamin deficiency	• Elder onset • Symmetrical distal sensorimotor neuropathy • History of alcoholism	1. Axonal degeneration with regeneration 2. Segmental demyelination with remyelination (rare)

(Continued)

Table 30.1 Other common peripheral neuropathies. *(Continued)*

Neuropathic disease	Causes	Clinical features	Microscopic features
Giant axonal neuropathy (GAN)	ARD associated with GAN mutation on Ch.16q23 encodes gigaxonin protein. It could occur as sporadic.	• Child-onset • Gait ataxia • Cognitive delay • Symmetrical distal sensorimotor neuropathy • MRI brain shows leukodystrophy-like feature	1. Giant axonal degeneration "swollen axons" 2. Axonal regeneration 3. Scattered OBFs 4. Distended axons in EM 5. Reduplicated basal laminae in EM 6. Filamentous accumulation in subaxolemmal area in EM
Amyloid neuropathy	**Familial**: Familial amyloid polyneuropathy (FAP); apolipoprotein A1 deposition due to Gly26Arg mutation **Non-familial**: *Primary*: Systemic AL-light chain *Secondary*: Serum protein A Others include: TTR type	• Adult-onset • May be asymptomatic • Slowly progressive • Symmetrical distal sensorimotor neuropathy • Painful parasthesia and muscle weakness • Autonomic dysfunction • Extra neurological features	1. Amyloid amorphous deposits in epineurium, perineurium, endoneurium, or within microvessels (red on Congo-red but light-green birefringence under polarized microscope) 2. Axonal degeneration with regeneration 3. Selective loss of unmyelinated fibers 4. Rare segmental demyelination 5. Amyloid fibrils in EM

(Continued)

Table 30.1 Other common peripheral neuropathies. (Continued)

Neuropathic disease	Causes	Clinical features	Microscopic features
Toxic neuropathy	**Sensory affection**: Cisplatin, ethambutol, isoniazid, tacrolimus, amiodaron, vincristine **Motor affection**: Chloroquine, colchicine	• Sensory neuropathy • Motor neuropathy • Medication or toxin history • History of psychiatric disease	1. Axonal degeneration 2. Selective loss of large myelinated fibers 3. Rare demyelination (tacrolimus, amiodaron) 4. Cellular lysosomal inclusions (amiodaron)

Abbreviations: PAN: polyarteritis nodosa. WG: Wegner granulomatosis. SLE: systemic lupus erythematosus. SD: Sjogren disease. IEL: internal elastic lamina. MCGUS: monoclonal gammopathy of unknown significance. ADD: autosomal dominant disease. ARD: autosomal recessive disease. CMTD: Charcot–Marie–Tooth disease. OBF: onion-bulb formation. Ig: Immunoglobulin. TTR: transthyretin. EM: electron microscopy. PMP22: peripheral myelin protein-2. MFN2: mitochondrial fusion protein-2. GDAP1: ganglioside-induced differentiation-associated protein 1. MRI: magnetic resonance imaging.

References

Adams D, Theaudin M, Cauqil C, et al. FAP neuropathy and emerging treatments. Curr Neurol Neurosci Rep. 2014; 14: 435.

Antoine JC, Mosnier JF, Absi L, et al. Carcinoma associated paraneoplastic peripheral neuropathies in patients with and without antionconeural antibodies. J Neurol Neurosurg Psychiatry. 1991; 67: 7–14

Arnold R, Kwai NCG, Krishnan AV. Mechanisms of axonal dysfunction in diabetic and uraemic neuropathies. Clin Neurophysiol. 2013; 124: 2079–2090.

Bailey RO, Ritaccio AL, Bishop MB, Wu AY. Benign monoclonal IgA gammopathy associated with polyneuropathy and dysautonomia. Acta Neurol Scand. 1986; 73: 574–580.

Behse F, Buchthal F. Alcoholic neuropathy: clinical, electrophysiological and biopsy findings. Ann Neurol. 1977; 2: 95–110.

Benstead TJ, Kuntz NL, Miller RG, Daube JR. The electrophysiologic profile of Dejerine-Sottas disease (HSMN-III). Muscle Nerve. 1990; 13: 586–592.

Berciano J, Combarros O, Figols J, et al. Hereditary motor and sensory neuropathy type II. Clinicopathological study of a family. Brain. 1986; 109: 897–914.

Bird SJ, Brown MJ. The clinical spectrum of diabetic neuropathy. Semin Neurol. 1996; 16: 115–122.

Blancas-Mejia LM, Ramirez-Alvarado M. Systemic amyloidosis. Annu Rev Biochem. 2013; 82: 745–774.

Bomont P, Cavalier L, Blondeau F, et al. The gene encoding gigaxonin, a new member of the cytoskeletal BTB/kelch repeat family is mutated in giant axonal neuropathy. Nat Genet. 2000; 26: 370–374.

Bouche P, Leger JM, Travers MA, et al. Peripheral neuropathy in systemic vasculitis: clinical and electrophysiologic study of 22 patients. Neurology. 1986; 36: 1598–1602.

Bradley WG, Lassman LP, Pearce GW, Walton JN. The neuromyopathy of vincristine in man. Clinical, electrophysiological and pathological studies. J Neurol Sci. 1970; 10: 107–131.

Camdessanch JP, Antoine JC, Honnorat J, et al. Paraneoplastic peripheral neuropathy associated with anti-Hu antibodies: a clinical and electrophysiological study of 20 patients. Brain. 2002; 125: 166–175.

Cavaletti G, Petruccioli MG, Crespi V, et al. A clinicopathological and followup study of 10 cases of essential type II cryoglobulinemic neuropathy. J Neurol Neurosurg Psychiatry. 1990; 53: 886–889.

Charness ME, Morady F, Scheinman MM. Frequent neurologic toxicity associated with amiodarone therapy. Neurology. 1984; 34: 669–671.

Chowdhury SKR, Smith DR, Fernyhough P. The role of aberrant mitochondrial bioenergetics in diabetic neuropathy. Neurobiol Dis. 2013; 51: 56–65.

Collins MP, Arnold WD, Kissel JT. The neuropathies of vasculitis. Neurol Clin. 2013; 31: 557–595.

Dalakas MC, Cunningham G. Characterization of amyloid deposits in biopsies of 15 patients with "sporadic" (non-familial or plasma cell dyscrasic) amyloid polyneuropathy. Acta Neuropathol. 1986; 69: 66–72.

Diaz-Arrastia R, Younger DS, Hair L. et al. Neurolymphomatosis: a clinicopathologic syndrome re-emerges. Neurology. 1992; 42: 1136–1141.

Florica B, Aghdassi E, Su J, et al. Peripheral neuropathy in patients with systemic lupus erythematosus. Semin Arthritis Rheum. 2011; 41: 203–211.

Gastaut JL, Pellissier JF. Neuropathie au cisplatine, etude Clinique electrophysiologique et morphologique. Rev Neurol. 1984; 141: 614–626.

Hanyu N, Ikeda S, Nakadai A, et al. Peripheral nerve pathological findings in familial amyloid polyneuropathy: a correlative study of proximal sciatic nerve and sural nerve lesions. Ann Neurol. 1989; 25: 340–350.

Hawke SHB, Davies L, Pamphlett YP, et al. Vasculitic neuropathy. A clinical and pathological study. Brain. 1991; 114: 2175–2190.

Hellmann DB, Laing TJ, Petri M, et al. Mononeuritis multiplex: the yield of evaluation for occult rheumatic diseases. Medicine. 1988; 67: 145–153.

Horwich MS, Cho L, Porro RS, Posner JB. Subacute sensory neuropathy: a remote effect of carcinoma. Ann Neurol. 1977; 2: 7–19.

Johansen P, Leegaard OF. Peripheral neuropathy and paraproteinemia: an immunohistochemical and serologic study. Clin Neuropathol. 1985; 4: 99–104.

Johnson PC, Brendel K, Meezan E. Human diabetic perineurial cell basement membrane thickening. Lab Invest. 1981; 44: 265–270.

Konishi T, Saida K, Ohnishi A, Nishitani H. Perineuritis in mononeuritis multiplex with cryoglobulinemia. Muscle Nerve. 1982; 5: 173–177.

Kretzschmar HA, Berg BO, Davis RL. Giant axonal neuropathy: a neuropathological study. Acta Neuropathol. 1987; 73: 138–144.

Lie JT. Systemic and isolated vasculitis. A rational approach to classification and pathologic diagnosis. Pathol Annu. 1989; 24: 25–114.

Luegetti M, Conte A, Montano N. Clinical and pathological heterogeneity in a series of 31 patients with IgM-related neuropathy. J Neurol Sci. 2012; 319: 75–80.

Naka T, Yorifuji S, Fujimura H, et al. A case of paraneoplastic neuropathy with necrotizing arteritis localized in the peripheral nervous system. Rinsho Shinkeigaku. 1991; 4: 427–432.

Nemni R, Corbo M, Fazio R, et al. Cryoglobulinaemic neuropathy. A clinical, morphological and immunocytochemical study of 8 cases. Brain. 1988; 111: 541–552.

Nemni R, Corbo M, Fazio R, et al. Cryoglobulinaemic neuropathy. A clinical, morphological and immunocytochemical study of 8 cases. Brain. 1988; 111: 541–552.

Prasnoor M, Dimachkie MM, Barohn RJ. Diabetic neuropathy part 2 proximal and asymmetric phenotypes. Neurol Clin. 2013; 31: 447–462.

Read DJ, Van Hegan RI, Matthews WB. Peripheral neuropathy and benign IgG paraproteinemia. J Neurol Neurosurg Psychiatry. 1978; 41: 215–298.

Sima AAF, Nathaniel V, Bril V, et al. Histopathological heterogeneity of neuropathy in insulin-dependent and non-insulin dependent diabetics and demonstration of axoglial dysjunction in human diabetic neuropathy. J Clin Invest. 1988; 81: 349–364

Takeuchi H, Takahashi M, Kang J, et al. Ethambutol neuropathy: clinical and electroneuromyographic studies. Folia Psychiatr Neurol Jpn. 1980; 34: 45–55.

Vital A, Lagueny A, Ferrer X, et al. Sarcoid neuropathy: clinicopathological study of 4 new cases and review of the literature. Clin Neuropathol. 2008; 27: 96–105.

Vital A, Vital C, Julien J, et al. Polyneuropathy associated with IgM monoclonal gammopathy: immunological and pathological study in 31 patients. Acta Neuropathol. 1989; 79: 160–167.

Younger DS, Rosoklija G, Hays AP, et al. Diabetic peripheral neuropathy: a clinicopathologic and immunohistochemical analysis of sural nerve biopsies. Muscle Nerve. 1996; 19: 722–727.

Italicized and **bold** pages refer to figures and tables respectively.

Index